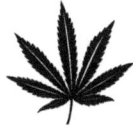

ENDORSEMENTS

I worked closely with Angie during the grand opening of Oakland County's first provisioning center. Its success is the direct result of her dedication and passion for the patients. Angie's persistent focus on patient safety and education sets her apart from the profit-driven businesses that dominate the market. She is the first person in-the-know on new discoveries in the field, always up to date on this ever-changing industry. As a patient, I would be hard-pressed to find a more compassionate and knowledgeable caregiver. As a colleague, her professionalism and mission-oriented drive are second to none. —*Ryan Schuler, Corpsman Veteran*

Angie is one of my go-to sources within the cannabis industry. Her knowledge and passion for cannabis put her in an elite class of individuals within the Michigan cannabis industry. Even I, someone who is knowledgeable about cannabis, seem to always learn something new from her when we talk. She has a great understanding of how the ECS works with cannabinoids/terpenes, and knows how to make appropriate recommendations for products and dosage. Angie and her work inspire me to learn more about cannabis, and I feel lucky to have a working relationship with her. —*Steve Scott, Craft Hemp Company*

Angie has all the knowledge and the expertise that a patient and a business could, and would, ever need. And when it comes to caregiving, well, I know from experience how kind and patient she is and that she gives 110% for her patients! She's definitely a team player and the kindest person I know. —*Sherry Hoover, Retired Beaumont Nurse/Cancer Patient*

Angie was instrumental in helping me understand how cannabis is used in the human body to heal itself. She helped me to understand its role in reaching homeostasis, essential to healing within our own body cannabinoid system. Yes, who knew we had a cannabinoid system! Angie does, and her knowledge is outstanding. She has a thorough knowledge from A-Z, from strains to terpenes, Cancer to Lyme—all facets of healing with cannabis. Not only is her expertise invaluable, but Angie goes above and beyond for her clients, specific to their individual health crisis. My particular cancer is quite rare, and Angie went out of her way to investigate/research cannabis in relation to my particular case in order to provide me with as much information and guidance as possible. She is as passionate as she is knowledgeable, and I highly recommend Angie to anyone who is on a healing journey. She is a wealth of information and a wonderful educator. She will always have your best interest at heart, and she will always have your back. I am truly grateful for her care, her compassion, her expertise, and I consider myself fortunate to have her in my healing journey. I am indebted to her genuine care and dedication, and proud to now also call her friend. —*Grateful survivor, thankful thriver Michelle*

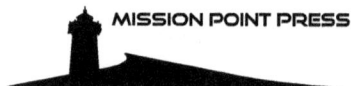

MISSION POINT PRESS

Published by Mission Point Press
2554 Chandler Rd.
Traverse City, MI 49696
(231) 421-9513
www.MissionPointPress.com

ISBN: 978-1-961302-13-6
Library of Congress Control Number: 2023915508
Printed in the United States of America

POT
for the
PEOPLE

The plant, the people, and the shop policies of cannabis

Angie Roullier

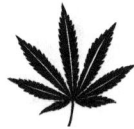

TABLE of CONTENTS

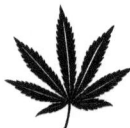

DISCLAIMER

Sometimes, it's easier to say what something isn't, as opposed to what it is. So, now I will tell you what this book isn't, and what I won't do.

What you will not get from this book is medical advice, as I have had zero medical training. All of the science included comes with direct links to the research supporting my statements and methods. I implore you to have very candid conversations with your doctors prior to starting a cannabis regimen. Drug interactions and certain cannabis compounds could do more harm than good. Cannabis is not for everyone.

You will also not get legal advice, as I have had zero legal training. Any mention of laws comes with direct links to where I get my information from. The purpose of this book is only to aid anyone interested in learning more about the products, the science behind medicating with cannabis, and the occasional nod to the cannabis culture. (I see no reason why someone cannot partake in marijuana for its potential medicinal benefits, and enjoy the plant-induced giggles at the very same time.)

You will find that I use several different terms when I talk about the plant and its users. I do this because this is the language of the people, but I will also introduce the proper terminology in hopes of aiding in the evolution of our industry. This book contains the fundamentals of cannabis and is made for easy reading so that everyone can understand and relate. And anyone who knows me personally knows that I use curse words like a comma. But for the most part I have restrained my language within these pages for the sensitivity of the masses. But you will find, on occasion, that my potty mouth shines through. What can I say, I enjoy colorful language.

You won't find specific recommendations for specific medical conditions in these pages—again I am not medically trained in any way—but I will offer references for research-based information and my opinions based upon said research for you to make your own educated decisions.

Brand endorsements are nowhere to be found in this book. But I will present resources on the different types of products, and ways to use cannabis, so you may be educated on how and what you might take for your own personal condition.

I will not name names of the people and places I have worked with, or at. In fact, all of the names have been changed in my personal stories to snub the egos of the guilty, to honor HIPAA laws, and to cover my own backside (plus, snitches get stitches). I admit that my memories may be different than those I speak about within these pages. And some of the stories are a mix of different people, making those stories technically fiction. I will apologize in advance for any offense or misrepresentations. I am here to do no harm, educate others with my experiences, and give you my knowledge the best way I know how.

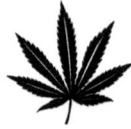

INTRODUCTION

Why write this book? Do we really need another opinion on this ever-evolving industry? Yes, I believe we do. We need one for the regular Joe. By a regular Jane.

Whether you call it marijuana, pot, weed, cannabis, or any of the dozens of other names for this ancient plant, it simply isn't going anywhere. Hell, this little plant was even deemed an "essential business" during the pandemic. As I write this, 39 states in our great country have some type of medical marijuana program, and 23 also allow for recreational adult use or have decriminalized it.[1] It's safe to say that cannabis is here to stay, and I have found that the vast majority of people in the aforementioned states have very basic questions when it comes to cannabis and how it works in "real life."

I'm a big fan of encouraging people to over-educate themselves when it comes to self-medicating with cannabis. Credible scientific research and personal responsibility are where it's at when it comes to using this plant as medicine. Over the past 12 years I have had thousands of people cross my path looking to cannabis for help with physical, mental, and/or emotional conditions. I have seen cannabis do wonders for so many of these people and I have seen it do absolutely nothing for others. Cannabis is not for everyone. Cannabis is not a cure-all, a magic bullet, or the last medicine you'll ever take. But what it may have is the potential to help. Naturally.

So, the questions still remain. Who can it help and who can it harm? Is there a difference between taking drops and eating a gummy? How is it possible that it can work for so many different things? Unfortunately, these questions are not being addressed properly by everyone, from doctors to the retail staff in our pot shops.

There is a huge disconnect between the ever-evolving research and getting the results to the actual consumer at the counter. But these answers are out there, it's just that most of it is not in plain English, nor is it all in one spot. I'm here to help sort some of it out for you with history, science, and stories from my interactions with medical marijuana patients, vendors, shop owners, and scientists. I encourage you to take a deeper dive into the subjects that interest you, because I am just scratching the surface here folks.

This is not one of those books that will demonize cannabis, nor will it put it on a pedestal. I am here to tell you about the encouraging research findings, how it works and how it doesn't, potential harmful interactions and, hopefully, I can squash some of the nonsense people believe surrounding this ancient plant.

I want to thank you in advance for being open-minded enough to take the time to learn about the plant that has both started wars and ended suffering. So, for everyone from my local pharmacist and city council members to the shameless birthday suit-parading senior in the women's locker room who have asked, "Why don't we know these things? Why isn't this information out there just like you explained it?" my hope is that the following pages will do exactly that. Happy learning folks!

---

[1] https://cannigma.com/us-states-where-cannabis-is-legal/

PROHIBITION

"If people let the government decide what foods they eat and what medicines they take, their bodies will soon be in as sorry a state as are the souls of those who live under tyranny."
– Thomas Jefferson

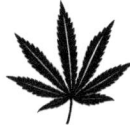

Oh, how I wish I could leave politics completely out of this book. I simply do not have the stomach for it. But alas, politics is so interwoven with this plant's history, present, and future, that if I ignored it completely, I would be doing you a huge disservice. So, I will go over it as quickly as I can so that we can get to the beauty and bewilderment that is the cannabis plant.

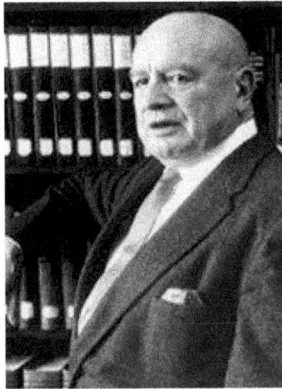

Harry J. Anslinger

This guy (insert heavy eye roll). Harry Anslinger had a pretty heavy hand in the banning of cannabis in the United States, even though he had been quoted saying that the notion that cannabis can make you violent was an "absurd fallacy." But that was before he needed job security.

In 1930, Anslinger was the first commissioner of the Federal Bureau of Narcotics, which is now known as the DEA, and stayed in control for 32 years. But since the prohibition of alcohol was falling apart, having been repealed in 1933, he had to find another "cause" to earn his keep with our federal government. The possession of heroin and cocaine, which were both banned in 1914, simply did not drum up enough business to protect him from the chopping block.

So Anslinger headed out, armed with only a fist full of articles from the 1920s (over a decade old at this point), claiming violent acts were caused by marijuana, beginning his crusade to outlaw cannabis to justify his existence.

But Anslinger ran into a little problem called science. When gathering 30 scientists to tell him what he wanted to hear, all but one reported that they couldn't find the violent behavioral claims he was looking for. In true thug fashion, Anslinger took the theory of the only guy willing to tell him what he needed to hear—that cannabis should be banned because it was evil—and ran to the newspapers with it. Of course, in the words of Don Henley, "we all know that crap is king," and unsurprisingly the press ran with the story.

———

The second act of his tall tale added fierce bigotry to the mix. Knowing that people were quick to judge and tag both Black and Mexican people for absolutely anything society found distasteful, Anslinger used that bigotry to his advantage. Some of the flat-out garbage that came out of his mouth were: "Reefer makes darkies think they are as good as white men," "Marijuana influences Negroes to look white people in the eye, step on white men's shadows and look at white women twice," and my favorite, "you smoke a joint and you're likely to kill your brother." I do not know about you, but smoking a joint *keeps* me from killing my brother.

Because of the ignorant racism of the day, Anslinger chose to utilize the Mexican spelling of marijuana, which replaced the "j" with an "h" to give it more attachment to the Mexicans he was scapegoating. There is a misconception that Anslinger and the publish-

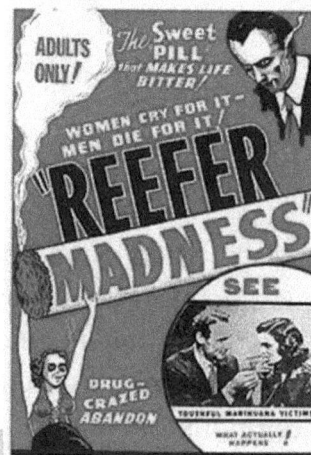

One cannot talk about Anslinger, especially a cannabis enthusiast, and not mention the overly comical propaganda of the 1936 flick *Reefer Madness*. The film was originally funded by a church under the title *Tell your Children* (also *Doped Youth* and *The Burning Question*) and was presented to parents as a matter of morals regarding the evils of cannabis.[3]

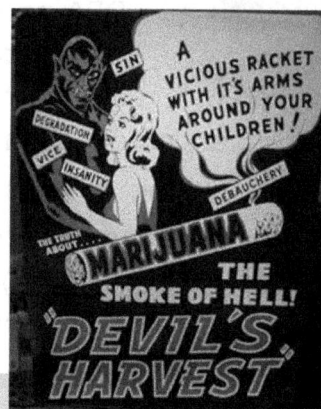

With more support from Hearst, the series continued to bombard the general public with savage tales such as *The Devil's Harvest, Assassins of Youth,* and *Marihuana Girl.* Today, these propaganda posters are cult classics and grace many a wall, my office included.[4]

ing monster William Randolph Hearst came up with this spelling, which is simply not true, as it had been a part of the Mexican pharmacopeia way, way before Anslinger snatched it up and made it a dirty word.[2] I'm honestly not surprised that he couldn't come up with any original ideas, as big entities run by small men rarely do. But as I write this, many governments still spell it with an "h" in their laws, and it is the reason you will hear people say that regardless of the spelling, the word marijuana is racist.

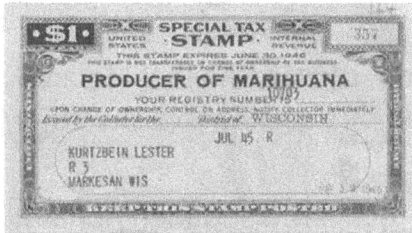

Marihuana Tax Act of 1937

In 1937, Anslinger's efforts paid off in the form of the Marihuana Tax Act, outlawing all things cannabis. The act removed cannabis from our pharmacopeia and required doctors and pharmacists to register and pay a fee to prescribe cannabis as medicine. Sound familiar? But as you can imagine, this caused the rate of prescriptions for cannabis to fall through the floor. This forced doctors to use other drugs, mostly opium-derived, for the treatment of their patients in pain.

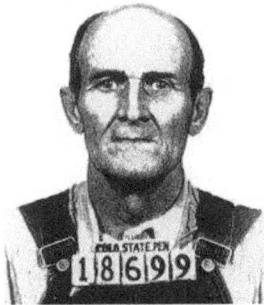

Not long after, the first arrests occurred under the new policy, with Denver City police and the Federal Bureau of Narcotics busting Samuel Caldwell for dealing and Moses Baca for possession. They were charged with not paying the marijuana tax under the new federal law. Baca was sentenced to 18 months, and Caldwell got slammed with a four-year stretch at Leavenworth Penitentiary. In the words of Ron Burgundy, "well, that escalated quickly."[5]

Hemp for Victory

The *Hemp for Victory* movie was produced by the US Department of Agriculture and released in 1942. Its purpose was to encourage farmers to grow as much hemp as they could for the war effort, as the other imported industrial fibers were in short supply. The movie showed the history of how hemp is grown, processed, and manufactured into rope, sails, and cordage.

[2]https://www.higherlearninglv.co/post/cannabis-vs-marijuana-debate-richard-rose-comments
[3]https://www.cnbs.org/cannabis-101/cannabis-prohibition/
[4]https://www.cbsnews.com/news/harry-anslinger-the-man-behind-the-marijuana-ban/
[5]https://en.wikipedia.org/wiki/Marihuana_Tax_Act_of_1937

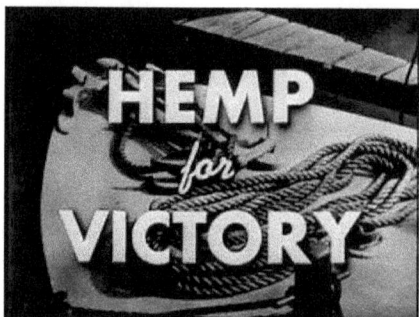

The Marihuana Tax Act of 1937 was lifted for a short time during World War II to allow for the manufacturing of hemp fiber for ropes for the US Navy. Once hemp did his patriotic duty, he was once again deemed illegal.

But even though this plant was requested by way of a government public campaign, the film was not widely known before 1989. In fact, the US government denied ever having made such a film! Both the US Department of Agriculture and our Library of Congress informed everyone that inquired about the picture that no such film was ever produced by the USDA, or any other branch of the government for that matter.

Yet low and behold, two VHS copies were in fact recovered and then donated to the Library of Congress on May 19th, 1989, by Maria Farrow, Carl Packard, and Jack Herer. May wonders never cease![6]

———

The cherry picking of evidence continued with the brushing off of the LaGuardia Report in 1944, in which the New York Academy of Medicine had run an extensive report and found that use of marijuana did not induce violence, insanity, or sex crimes, or lead to addiction or other drug use; and yet the hypocrisy just kept coming.[7]

The next push was in the form of the Boggs Act of 1952, which tacked on a minimum sentence of two to ten years and a fine of up to $20,000 for your first possession offense.[8] Following this, the Narcotic Control Act of 1956 changed the Internal Revenue Code of 1954 and the Narcotic Drugs Import and Export Act so they could more "effectively" control narcotics, including marijuana.[9]

Part of the act was ruled unconstitutional in 1969, in Lear v. United States, because of a direct violation of our Fifth Amendment rights. A person could not

---

[6]https://en.wikipedia.org/wiki/Hemp_for_Victory
[7]https://www.law.du.edu/documents/marijuana-summit/La-Guardia-Report.pdf
[8]https://komornlaw.com/the-boggs-act-of-1951/
[9]https://www.unodc.org/unodc/en/data-and-analysis/bulletin/bulletin_1956-01-01_3_page005.html#s0001
[10]https://en.wikipedia.org/wiki/Marihuana_Tax_Act_of_1937

apply for a tax stamp without cutting their own throat. The answer from Congress was the Controlled Substance Act, which was attached to the Comprehensive Drug Abuse Prevention and Control Act of 1970. This repealed the 1937 act.[10]

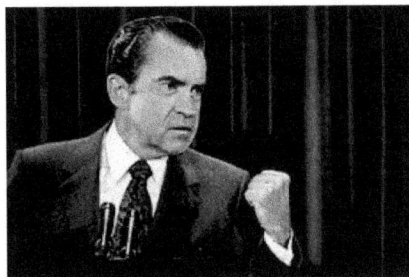

Cannabis Becomes a Schedule 1 Drug

The Controlled Substance Act of 1970 was signed by President Nixon, which combined all prior existing federal drug laws into one single statute. And in June 1971, Nixon officially declared a "War on Drugs," stating that drug abuse was "public enemy number one."

Under this act a "schedule" was created to rank substances by their medical value and their potential for abuse. Cannabis found itself lumped in with heroin, LSD, and ecstasy as a Schedule I drug.[11]

One of the most powerful statements against cannabis prohibition came, iron-ically, from one of the DEA's own Chief Administrative Law Judges, Francis Young. Young, after lengthy hearings regarding the usefulness of the herb in 1988, stated, "Marijuana, in its natural form, is one of the safest therapeutically active substances known. It would be unreasonable, arbitrary, and capricious for the DEA to continue to stand between those sufferers and the benefits of this substance …."

Unfortunately, despite this strong official opinion, the DEA did not implement his ruling and allowed the rescheduling of cannabis, citing a procedural technicality.[12]

Patent 6630507

Again, being labeled as a Schedule I drug means that there isn't any currently accepted medical value, and that it has a high potential for abuse; according to this ranking system, the US government sees cocaine, oxycodone, and fentanyl as having greater medicinal value and being less risky for potential abuses.[13]

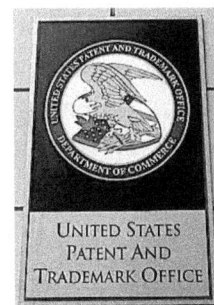

UNITED STATES
PATENT AND
TRADEMARK OFFICE

---

[10] https://en.wikipedia.org/wiki/Marihuana_Tax_Act_of_1937

[11] https://www.encyclopedia.com/history/encyclopedias-almanacs-transcripts-and-maps/controlled-substanc-es-act-1970

[12] https://norml.org/news/2013/09/05/25-years-ago-dea-s-own-administrative-law-judge-ruled-cannabis-should-be-reclassified-under-federal-law/

[13] https://www.dea.gov/drug-information/drug-scheduling

But did you know that up until April 21st, 2019,[14] the US government held the patent on certain compounds found in the cannabis plant for their potential medicinal values? They did not "own" the entire plant, nobody can, but their patent includes the potential use of "non-psychoactive" (wrong word, but we'll keep going) cannabinoids to protect the brain from damage, and provide treatments for Alzheimer's, Parkinson's, HIV, and dementia.[15][16]

Hmmm ....

So, does cannabis have medicinal value or not? If you are a government-influenced pharmaceutical company, the answer is yes. There are several drugs out there that use cannabinoids (mostly man-made synthetics) for the treatment of epilepsy and for the side effects of chemotherapy. But if you're just a regular Joe, the answer is no, unless you are prescribed one of the drugs mentioned above.

I'll let you choose the adjectives to describe the situation.

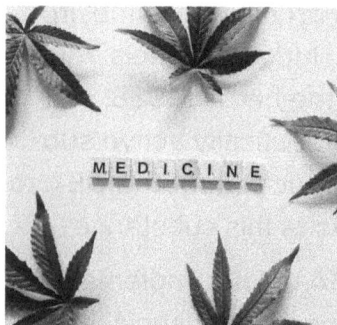

Big Pharma

A group of economists has put forth new research that estimates that the legalization of both medical and recreational cannabis over the past two and a half decades has cost pharmaceutical companies billions (with a "b") in lost sales. And if (when) cannabis is made completely legal nationwide, it would degrade the value of their stocks by over 10%.

Sorry. Not Sorry.

As more and more states break the chains of prohibition in our great country, researchers are finding some remarkable, interesting, and healthier changes to the population's choices in medications. There have been several studies that show a significant drop in opioid scripts after medical cannabis was allowed in a state. There is also a link between having access to medical marijuana and a lower number of general scripts being filled.[17]

---

[14]https://mmjhealth.com/everything-you-should-know-about-the-cannabis-patent/.
[15]https://uspatent6630507.com/
[16]https://patents.google.com/patent/US6630507B1/en
[17]https://newatlas.com/health-wellbeing/cannabis-legalization-us-big-pharma-billions-drug-sales

---

But as you can imagine, this is not going to stop Big Pharma from trying to regain their control. In fact, they have been working on it for years.

———

There have been a few approved drugs using synthetic cannabinoids over the past few years. Dronabinol (Marinol®) and Nabilone (Cesamet®) were made to combat nausea and stimulate some sort of an appetite for patients struggling through chemotherapy treatments and those with wasting diseases, such as AIDS patients. There is also Nabiximols (Sativex), a synthetic, cannabis-based mouth spray formulated for dealing with the spasticity and nerve pain from such diseases as Multiple Sclerosis. This medication combines both THC and CBD cannabinoids and is available in the UK, Canada, and a few other European countries.

And then there is the first FDA-approved, cannabis-based drug, Epidiolex.[18] This is a liquid medication containing CBD isolate to aid in combating two rare forms of childhood epilepsy: Dravet syndrome and Lennox-Gastaut syndrome. And like a backhanded compliment, it was made into a Schedule V drug that will run you around $32,500 a year.[19] Let me remind you yet again that the law of the land still stands by its Schedule I label on cannabis as not having any medicinal value.[20]

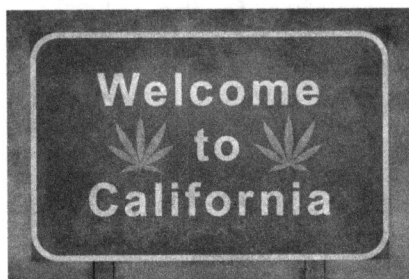

Prop 215

Let's get away from regression and get into some progression by flashing forward to 1996 and the west side of our nation. The Compassionate Use Act of 1996 is a law in California allowing the possession and use of medical cannabis. The law passed on November 5th, 1996, with 55.6% of voters in favor. This caused quite a clash on the topic of a state's rights versus our federal government, as this was the first ballot initiative passed at the state level.[21]

---

[18]https://www.fda.gov/news-events/public-health-focus/fda-and-cannabis-research-and-drug-approval-pro-cessThis

[19]https://naturebyscience.com/how-much-does-epidiolex-cost-the-cost-may-shock-you/

[20]https://nida.nih.gov/publications/research-reports/marijuana/marijuana-safe-effective-medicine

[21]https://en.wikipedia.org/wiki/1996_California_Proposition_215

Even though cannabis is still federally illegal, as of June 2022, there are 39 states, including the District of Columbia and Puerto Rico, that have some variation of a medical marijuana program. Out of these states, 23 of them have total adult-use programs or have decriminalized cannabis. This freight train of change shows no signs of slowing down, and everyone involved, from scientists and doctors to the novice consumer, should know the basics of cannabis use and the laws in your area.[22]

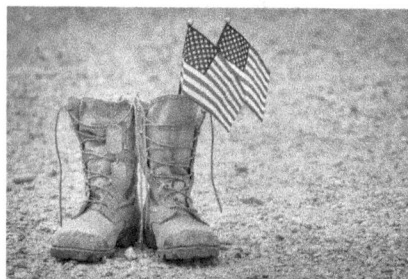

Dr. Sue Sisley
Our newfound industry has some true warriors that are using their passion, intelligence, and backbones to force our country to play fair when it comes to researching this plant.

Dr. Sue Sisley is one of these brawlers.[23]

Sue is a physician of internal medicine and psychiatry from Arizona and president of Scottsdale Research Institute. She has accomplished many milestones for cannabis and biotech more broadly, such as serving as a volunteer cannabis medical director for over 40 state operating licenses and continually fighting for quality, realistic cannabis samples in order to conduct clinical trials. She serves as the principal investigator for the only FDA-approved randomized controlled trial. In this trial, she is looking at the safety and efficiency of inhaled cannabis flower in relationship to combat veterans and PTSD.[24]

But these accomplishments (and so many more) didn't come lightly to Sue. Anytime someone takes on the beast that is medical research in this country, they're bound to take the consequences on the chin.

In 2014, Sue received approval from the NIDA (National Institutes of Drug Addiction) to study the potential efficiency between cannabis and PTSD at the University of Arizona. She was then abruptly fired for it, just before getting a $2 million grant from the state of Colorado to study this relationship.[25]

---

[22]https://cannigma.com/us-states-where-cannabis-is-legal/
[23]https://www.trailblazerspresents.com/sue-sisley
[24]https://hiimr.humboldt.edu/sue-sisley
[25]https://www.cannabisbusinessexecutive.com/2016/07/politico-100/

And then she got dropped like a hot potato by another corporate oaf: Bank of America.

———

"Bank of America closes down account of Federally licensed cannabis researcher," Sue wrote on Twitter. "SRI conducts FDA approved controlled trials evaluating cannabis as medicine for treating pain/PTSD in military veterans & terminally ill patients, this TRAGICALLY shuts down our research."[26]

———

Even though the bank had issued her a letter, it did not give her any reasons, only that the choice to shut down the account was reached "after a careful review of your banking relationship." So, even though she had been banking with them for ten years because they were a federally OK'd "plant-touching" organization, she and her research were left swinging in the wind. The letter ended with, "this decision is final and won't be reconsidered,"[27] Nice, huh?

I was lucky enough to see Sue present at a symposium in Ann Arbor a few years back. She presented pictures of what the only government-sourced "product" looked like that she was expected to run her trial with. Let me tell you that it was the seedy, stemmy oregano from the days of acid-washed jeans and Aqua Net. As her research is based on realistic cannabis access for medical reasons, she knew this garbage was unacceptable.

There are those that will only push things past the outer limits when they have nothing left to lose. Sue is not one of these people. Risking more than we can ever know, she kept sprinting forward without looking back.

Only a few years ago, the University of Mississippi was the only one federally approved and licensed to grow cannabis for medical research in the U.S.

Since Sue is not one to just sit back and only take what is given to her (especially if it wasn't what she needed), she fought back. She sued the DEA in 2019 after getting the cold shoulder regarding her 2016 submitted application to "grow her own" marijuana for medical research purposes, due to the current poor quality of the plant available.

---

[26]https://va.org/news/boa-shuts-account-cannabis-research-firm
[27]https://www.cannabisbusinesstimes.com/news/bank-of-america-closes-account-cannabis-research-er-sue-sisley/

In true conquering fashion, Sue succeeded in landing a DEA Schedule I bulk manufacturer license. This victory of historical proportions not only ended the 52-year government monopoly on cannabis research, but now paves future roads for the private sector to grow cannabis flower for FDA-approved clinical trials.[28]

Sue knows that the place vets and cannabis meet is at the local pot shop; you have to go to where the people actually are in order to test what they have access to and what their preferred method of intake is. Our industry is truly lucky to have such an intelligent and empathetic lady fighting for cannabis—fighting for us.[29]

---

[28]https://www.cannabisbusinesstimes.com/news/groff-north-american-brings-private-sector-cannabis-to-us-market/

[29]https://www.trailblazerspresents.com/sue-sisley

PLANT

"The art of medicine consists of amusing the
patient while nature cures the disease."
— Voltaire

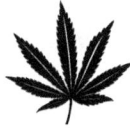

Disclaimer

We have only just begun the journey to fully understanding the natural chemicals of cannabis and the promise they may hold as plant-based medicine. Just thinking about not only the different independent compounds, but the endless combinations of these compounds, quite frankly makes my head hurt. Thankfully, there are those out there that have a true passion for such tasks and take it as far as they can on a daily basis.

—

As I will state several times throughout these pages, these are the very, very bare bones of what we know so far. And I am sure that there is an abundance of scientists and scholars alike that will say that I haven't explained the plant (or its effects) to its fullest extent. Of course, I haven't. I am not a scientist, and they don't even know all there is to know about the matter.

I want you to think of the following terms, definitions, and examples as if I am a senior in high school tutoring a 5th grader in English for the purpose of understanding verbs, adjectives, and proper nouns. Again, these are the bare bones as we currently know them.

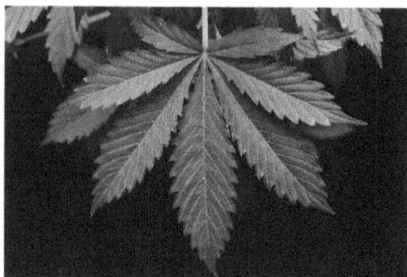

HEMP VS. MARIJUANA

We have all heard both terms when referencing cannabis, but what exactly is the difference between the two? Both come from Cannabis sativa L, but what separates them is partly genetics, and partly a matter of the law of the land. Let's start with genetics.

According to the hash museum, "'Cannabis' is the name given to the plant itself. 'Sativa' simply means 'sown' and is used to indicate the common or cultivated form of the plant. The 'L' refers to Carolus Linneaeus, the Swedish botanist who first gave this common yet celebrated herb its scientific classification in 1753.

Since then, two more main types of cannabis have been identified: Cannabis indica was classified in 1785 and Cannabis Ruderalis in 1924. Both are sub-species of the Cannabis sativa family, and the three types are distinguished by the different characteristics and traits they display."[30]

Think along the lines of the tomato plant. You can have Cherry, Roma, or Heirloom tomatoes. They are each different in size, acidity, and consistency, but at the end of the day they are all still tomatoes.

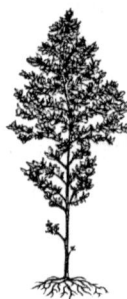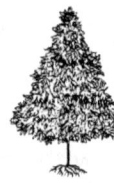

Sativa   Indica   Ruderalis

Hemp is generally bred for its industrial use in fiber, fuel, and food, while marijuana is grown for the medicinal value of its cannabinoids. Since the Farm Bill of 2018, the definition is that any cannabis plant that has more than 0.3% of THC is considered to be marijuana, and anything less is hemp. Imagine you are a hemp farmer that sells his harvest for fiber in the clothing industry, but for whatever reason the crop tests at 0.7% THC. This farmer now has acres of very illegal marijuana, and some very big problems.

---

[30]https://hashmuseum.com/en/cannabis-knowledge/cannabis-species/

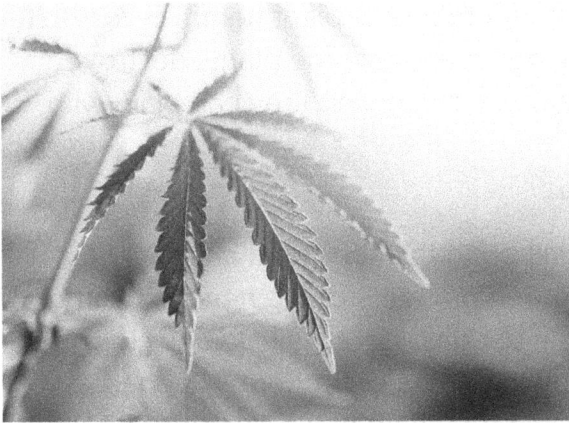

It turns out that cannabis is a superhero before it even leaves the dirt.

Cannabis is a bioaccumulator by nature. In fact, it is a hyperaccumulator, along with sunflowers and mustard plants. Cannabis has the capacity to absorb metals and other toxins from soil by drinking them in through their roots, where it is then moved and stored in their stems and leaves.

One of my favorite examples of this was an Italian sheep farmer that discovered in 2008 that his land had been poisoned by dioxin, a toxic chemical that is extremely difficult to break down once it is in the environment. Dioxin can cause cancer, reproductive and developmental problems, damage to the immune system, and can interfere with hormones.[31]

This toxin, known to be stored in the fatty tissue of animals, had been leaking from a large steel plant in the area, which prompted the Italian government to test this farmer's livestock for the contaminant. With the tests coming back positive, he was forced to slaughter his entire herd of 600 sheep.

Not willing to give up on his land, the farmer implemented the idea to plant hemp for its bioaccumulating skills in hopes that it would save his farm. Not only would the hemp rid his part of the planet of toxins in the dirt, but the garbage-grabbing crop could also be burned later as biofuel. Although time consuming, this method can provide a natural fuel source.[32]

But buyer beware, as this fact warrants caution. Yes, it's very cool that this plant can clean the dirt, but think about all of those toxins contained within a plant that may end up being harvested for human consumption (CBD). If the processor isn't careful, the heavy metals could (and sometimes do) make their way into that CBD tincture or gummy that you are so fond of. Always check the test results, better known as a COA (certificate of analysis), for any heavy metals.

---

[31] https://www.epa.gov/dioxin/learn-about-dioxin
[32] https://ecosciences.com/blog/health-and-lifestyle/hemp-can-clean-contaminated-soil/

On a positive note, I have heard of many farmers that plant hemp for the first couple of seasons to clean their own land, and then have the plants destroyed. After a few rounds of hemp, their dirt is squeaky clean, and they can plant with the confidence of a clean end product.

———

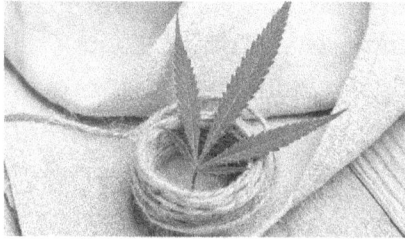

I couldn't bring this topic to a close without a nod to two true pioneers of the hemp industry. The first is a daughter to a New Jersey clothing designer by the name of Barbara Filippone, who is responsible for taking hemp fiber way beyond rope and grain sacks.

At the age of 17, she was working with Indian companies that were importing clothing to New York. She worked with designers and importers to properly showcase the beauty of hemp fabrics, and this in turn led her to the sweatshops in India. Upon witnessing the deplorable conditions that rendered its workers ill and rapidly aging from the exposure to the chemicals used to process the fabrics, Barbara looked for a better way.

The opportunity to continue her work beyond the factories of India came in the early 1990s, when she hitched her wagon to the company Earth Goods, and again in 2002 when she started her own company, EnviroTextiles, with the help of her daughter.

According to her interview with Jeremy Briggs at Hemp Frontiers, "EnviroTextiles has developed numerous 100%-hemp woven and knit fabrics and blends, including hemp/cotton, hemp/silk, and hemp/tencel (Hempcel®). They also supply yarn, fiber, and the highest quality hemp t-shirt offered today."

Her passions stem from what she witnessed in the sweatshops as well as her love of fabrics from her mother, and with those in mind, she has championed two equally important advancements. Firstly, she has created many industry changing processes for turning hemp fiber into fabric and is also setting the bar for eco-friendly, natural textiles by creating a new labeling system.

The other advancement takes her beyond the idea of "organic," into fibers that are raised with integrity, and by proxy leaving what returns to the earth clean.

[33]*https://therichardrosereport.com/hemp-textiles-og-barbara-filippone/*
[34]*https://hempfrontiers.com/hemp-fabric-pioneer-of-the-modern-era-barbara-filippone/*

Barbara believes that "Recycling is a temporary solution for something that we don't know how to dispose of." She's not wrong.[33][34]

The other crusader of hemp is Chris Boucher. It was a fateful day in 1990 when Chris found himself being asked by Jack Herer, the author of *The Emperor Wears No Clothes*, to sign a petition to legalize hemp, and his whole world changed. Not knowing what hemp really was, he asked Jack to explain it to him. Hours later, after going chapter by chapter through his book, Chris was inspired. "'Let's change the world. This is the greatest environmental product commodity ever grown." And it was American. "It was really the roots of America, how we were successful in commerce and global commerce and shipping and so forth and so on," Mr. Boucher said during a 2022 interview with Eric Hurlock.[35]

In those days you could only get your hemp from China, Poland, or Romania, so Chris took it upon himself to create an American-made resource. In 1994, with the USDA's blessing, Chris became the first person to legally grow hemp in the United States in decades. His meager crop of just a couple of acres was located in Brawley, California, at the USDA Research Station. But with or without permission, local narcotics agents soon came along and destroyed his first crop before he could harvest it.

As a true pioneer, Chris just kept plugging away. He co-founded the Hemp Industries Association (HIA), imported the first CBD oil into the United States, and co-wrote the legal opinion "Hemp CBD is legal in all 50 States" in 2012, which still influences legal battles today.[36]

However, cannabis history groupies be warned when striking up a conversation with this trailblazer. Mr. Boucher considers "industrial" to be a dirty word when applied to hemp. In the same interview, Chris goes on to explain his disdain for the term. "Well, because hemp started as an environmental movement. We wanted to clean up the soil. We could do the fiber, the fabrics and oil and food, and it was one of the best environmental crops we knew of compared to any other crop that existed. So a group of people, people that I knew, liked the name industrial. And to us, it sounded like a toxic, polluting name—industrial. It doesn't sound environmental."[37]

---

[35]*https://www.lancasterfarming.com/farming-news/hemp/podcast/chris-bouchers-thirty-year-journey-into-hemp/article_fc860fd0-09e0-11ed-a92c-ab67be154025.html*
[36]*https://www.farmtiva.com/about*
[37]*https://www.farmtiva.com/about*

CANNABINOIDS

By definition, "Cannabinoids, broadly speaking, are a class of biological compounds that bind to cannabinoid receptors. They are most frequently sourced from and associated with the plants of the Cannabis genus, including *Cannabis sativa*, *Cannabis indica*, and *Cannabis ruderalis*."[38]

Cannabinoids come in these three forms:
- *Phyto*cannabinoids – comes from the plant.
- *Endo*cannabinoids – your body makes them naturally.
- Synthetic Cannabinoids – man-made.

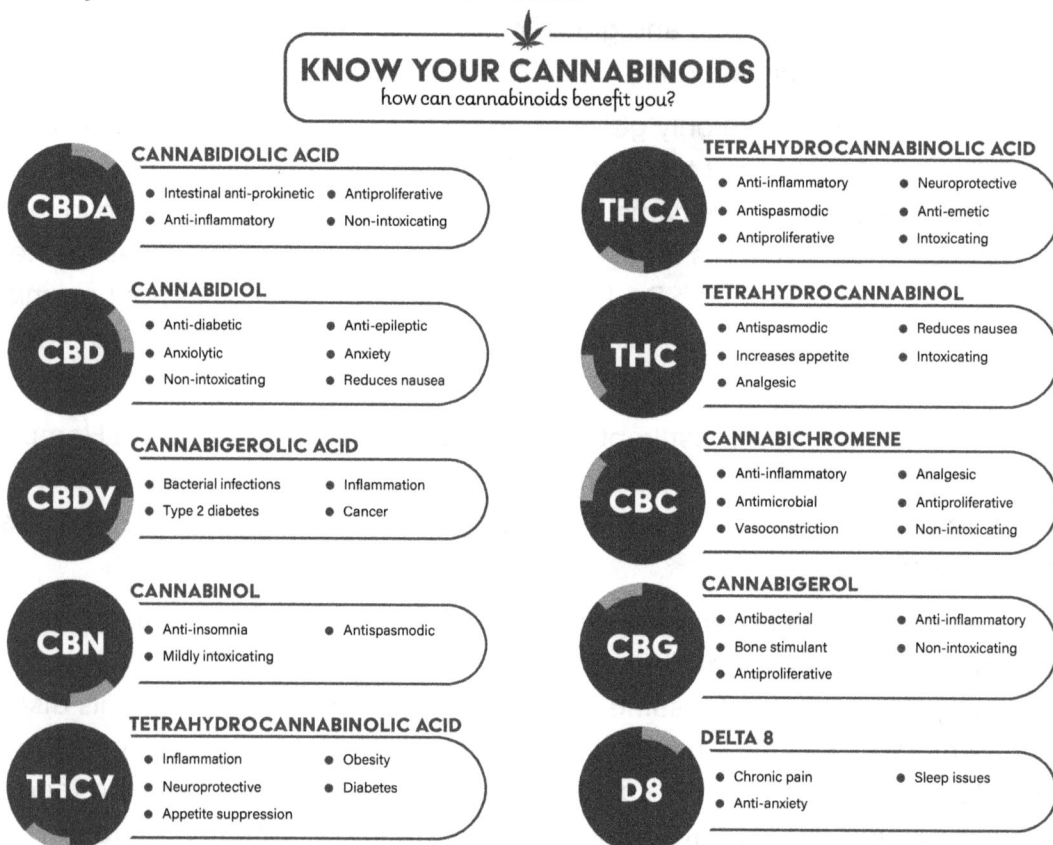

KNOW YOUR CANNABINOIDS
how can cannabinoids benefit you?

CBDA — CANNABIDIOLIC ACID
- Intestinal anti-prokinetic
- Anti-inflammatory
- Antiproliferative
- Non-intoxicating

CBD — CANNABIDIOL
- Anti-diabetic
- Anxiolytic
- Non-intoxicating
- Anti-epileptic
- Anxiety
- Reduces nausea

CBDV — CANNABIGEROLIC ACID
- Bacterial infections
- Type 2 diabetes
- Inflammation
- Cancer

CBN — CANNABINOL
- Anti-insomnia
- Mildly intoxicating
- Antispasmodic

THCV — TETRAHYDROCANNABINOLIC ACID
- Inflammation
- Neuroprotective
- Appetite suppression
- Obesity
- Diabetes

THCA — TETRAHYDROCANNABINOLIC ACID
- Anti-inflammatory
- Antispasmodic
- Antiproliferative
- Neuroprotective
- Anti-emetic
- Intoxicating

THC — TETRAHYDROCANNABINOL
- Antispasmodic
- Increases appetite
- Analgesic
- Reduces nausea
- Intoxicating

CBC — CANNABICHROMENE
- Anti-inflammatory
- Antimicrobial
- Vasoconstriction
- Analgesic
- Antiproliferative
- Non-intoxicating

CBG — CANNABIGEROL
- Antibacterial
- Bone stimulant
- Antiproliferative
- Anti-inflammatory
- Non-intoxicating

D8 — DELTA 8
- Chronic pain
- Anti-anxiety
- Sleep issues

Note: This graphic was updated on July 22, 2025 to correct information that was inaccurate in earlier printings. The publisher and author do not guarantee the accuracy of earlier versions and encourage readers to refer to this updated version for the most current information.

THC and CBD are considered to be "major" cannabinoids, while any others are considered to be "minor" or "rare" cannabinoids due to the low concentrations found in the plant. But much like the Cusack siblings, I believe that they are not getting the credit they deserve. Just because these cannabinoids are less

---

[38] https://www.ncbi.nlm.nih.gov/books/NBK556062/

abundant does not mean that they don't have their own roles to play.

(Since I struggle with saying the names of some of these cannabinoids, I have taken it upon myself to do my best in spelling out the pronunciations of the overly large and intimidating words.)

—

Let's take a look at the top ten cannabinoids and their pros and cons.

THC stands for Tetrahydrocannabinol (tetra-hydro-ka-nab-a-nall), is intoxicating, and can also be referred to as Delta 9 or D9. This is the cannabinoid that is notorious for the "high" people can feel when using cannabis.

My goodness, how so many people get all wound up over these three little letters. But THC, in moderation, is not such a bad guy after all. He's just misunderstood and often misused.

Potential beneficial effects of THC

| Chronic Pain | Glaucoma | Muscle Spasticity |
| Low Appetite | Nausea Issues | Sleep Issues |

THC also comes with both good and bad side effects. The undesirable ones can be overwhelming and even downright dangerous if a person consumes too much.[39]

Potential negative effects of THC

Coordination Problems	Delayed Reaction Times	
Dry Mouth	Anxiety	Dry/Red Eyes
Memory Loss	Intoxication	Increased Heart Rate

The cannabis plant does not make THC, but rather THCA, and it is up to humans and/or time to change it.

---

[39] *https://www.healthline.com/health/cbd-vs-thc#medical-benefits*

THCA stands for Tetrahydrocannabinolic Acid (tetra-hydro-ka-nab-in-o-lick), is nonintoxicating, and is the precursor to the ever-popular THC. So, in English, if you were to pluck a fresh bud from a flowering cannabis plant and pop it into your mouth, THCA is what you would get (among other things). Adding raw cannabis to your diet is becoming more popular, and I have to say I am a big admirer. For me personally, THCA feels like getting a shot of B12.

Now, if you hit the same bud with heat, you will be knocking off the "A" (acid form), leaving you with the intoxicating THC that we all know. This is called decarboxylation, or decarbing, for short. We will get into what temperatures the different cannabinoids can convert and/or cook off at later on. But until then, let's focus on what this nonintoxicating acid form of THC can do before you spark it.[40]

Potential beneficial effects of THCA

Inflammation   Epilepsy   Nausea

Potential negative effects of THCA

Jitters   Lack of Sleep

Can be unstable due to Conversion

---

[40]*https://www.projectcbd.org/medicine/dosing-thca-less-more*

CBD stands for Cannabidiol (canna-bid-dial), is nonintoxicating, and is the second most popular cannabinoid found in the cannabis plant. It is well known for offering therapeutic properties without the "high" that her big sister THC carries. The WHO (World Health Organization) reports, "In humans, CBD exhibits no effects indicative of any abuse or dependence potential … To date, there is no evidence of public health related problems associated with the use of pure CBD."[41]

Potential beneficial effects of CBD

| Anxiety | Chronic Pain | Inflammation |
| Sleep Issues | Nausea | Addiction |

This cannabinoid seems to be everywhere and promises to do everything. This is not the case. CBD should be treated like any other drug and requires your due diligence when considering taking CBD as medicine.

Potential negative effects of CBD

| Dry Mouth | Nausea | Drug Interactions |
| Diarrhea | Sleep Issues | |

Let's talk about the term "nonpsychoactive," and how it relates to cannabis. This always reminds me of the words of Inigo Montoya, "You keep using that word; I do not think it means what you think it means."

This term seems to be plastered everywhere from your local CBD shop to research papers to induce a feeling of consumer security and a harmless alternative to pharmaceuticals. It is meant to ease our minds that the compound and/or the product will not get us high. Although CBD and the other "nonpsychoactive" cannabinoids will not get you stoned in the traditional sense of the word, it is definitely influencing your brain.

---

[41]https://www.health.harvard.edu/blog/cannabidiol-cbd-what-we-know-and-what-we-dont-2018082414476
[42]https://medical-dictionary.thefreedictionary.com/psychoactive

---

By definition, psychoactive is "Possessing the ability to alter mood, anxiety, behavior, cognitive process or mental tension...."[42]

So therefore, caffeine and nicotine are a couple of other substances that are also considered to be psychoactive, yet these effects don't translate into being "stoned," as society sees it.

Those of us that are into the medical/science side of the cannabis industry prefer the more accurate term of "nonintoxicating." This verbiage sets a very clear distinction, not only between catching a buzz or not, but the effects it has on our brains as well.

CBDA, which stands for Cannabidiolic Acid (canna-bid-all-lick), is nonintoxicating and is considered to be a minor cannabinoid, having been first isolated in 1955. Just as THCA is the precursor to THC, CBDA is the precursor to CBD. It requires heat to drop the "A" and change the compound and its effects. CBDA + heat = CBD.

This little beauty has been shown to be 1000x more potent in reducing nausea than CBD and seems to play well with the other cannabinoids by enhancing their benefits.[43]

Potential beneficial effects of CBDA

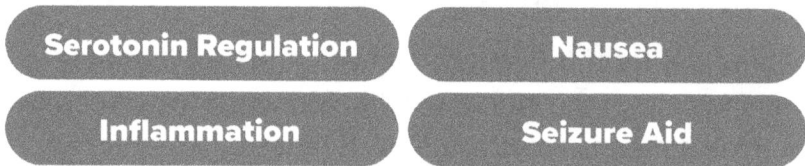

- Serotonin Regulation
- Nausea
- Inflammation
- Seizure Aid

Potential negative effects of CBDA

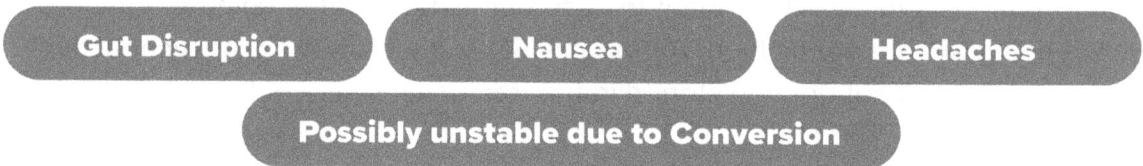

- Gut Disruption
- Nausea
- Headaches
- Possibly unstable due to Conversion

---

[43]https://www.ncbi.nlm.nih.gov/pmc/articles/PMC8669157/

CBN stands for Cannabinol (canna-bee-nall), is semi-intoxicating, and was initially isolated from Indian hemp in 1896, which made it the very first phytocannabinoid to be identified in cannabis. CBN is not made by the plant itself but is the end result of THC that has been degraded.

In plain English, this means that when your weed is exposed to air and light/heat over time, it turns into a completely new compound with different effects than the THC you started with.[44]

You will see more and more companies claim that CBN is the go-to for sleep, but the research is really scarce.[45]

There is, however, more evidence piling up about some other great benefits.

Potential beneficial effects of CBN

Chronic Pain — Appetite — Inflammation

Fibromyalgia — Immune Health

Potential negative effects of CBN[46]

Intoxication — Appetite Stimulant — Lack of Sleep

CBC stands for Cannabichromene (canna-bicker-mean), is nonintoxicating and is one of the most plentiful minor cannabinoids found in cannabis. In the 1980s, the anti-inflammatory effects of CBC were shown to be more effective than NSAIDs (nonsteroidal anti-inflammatory drug), such as ibuprofen or aspirin.

Like some of the other interactive behaviors of cannabinoids, CBC works better as an anti-inflammatory when mixed with THC than when either cannabinoid is used alone.[47]

---

[44] https://www.ncbi.nlm.nih.gov/pmc/articles/PMC8669157/

[45] https://www.ncbi.nlm.nih.gov/pmc/articles/PMC8612407/

[46] These negative effects may be from CBN channeling its THC ancestor and producing a watered-down version of its effects. https://www.ncbi.nlm.nih.gov/pmc/articles/PMC8669157/ [47] https://medical-dictionary.thefreedictionary.com/psychoactive

[47] Walsh KB, McKinney AE, Holmes AE. Minor Cannabinoids: Biosynthesis, Molecular Pharmacology and Potential Therapeutic Uses. Front Pharmacol. 2021 Nov 29;12:777804. doi: 10.3389/fphar.2021.777804. PMID: 34916950; PMCID: PMC8669157.

Potential beneficial effects of CBC

Migranes	Bone Strength	Inflammation

Neuroprotection	Tumors

Potential negative effects of CBC

Dizzy	Dry Mouth	Nausea

CBGA stands for Cannabigerolic Acid (canna-bige-er-o-lick), is nonintoxicating, and is considered to be the mother of all cannabinoids, as it is the precursor to THCA, CBDA, and CBCA. Since the acid form will naturally decarb (convert) over time, it is rare to find CBGA concentrations in fully grown cannabis plants.[48]

Imagine plucking an unripe green tomato. This is the stage, in a cannabis plant, where you will find CBGA. If you leave it be and let it continue to mature, the once-CBGA will have converted to THCA by the time you are ready to harvest.

Potential beneficial effects of CBGA

Inflammation	Cancer

Bacterial Infections	Type 2 Diabetes

Potential negative effects of CBGA

Diarrhea	Tiredness

Changes in Appetite

[48]Walsh KB, McKinney AE, Holmes AE. Minor Cannabinoids: Biosynthesis, Molecular Pharmacology and Potential Therapeutic Uses. Front Pharmacol. 2021 Nov 29;12:777804. doi: 10.3389/fphar.2021.777804. PMID: 34916950; PMCID: PMC8669157.

CBG stands for Cannabigerol (canna-bidge-err-all), is nonintoxicating, and is the precursor to THC and CBD. Those with cancer often experience a lack of appetite, but CBG offers an alternative to the buzz-inducing effects of THC by also stimulating hunger which results in an increase of food ingested.

Not surprisingly, CBG taken in whole-plant preparations was found to be more effective than the isolated form of CBG.[49]

Potential beneficial effects of CBG

- Inflammation
- Cancer
- Neuroprotectant
- Appetite

** There wasn't any sound research to warrant a slide on the negatives of CBG.**

THCV, or Tetrahydrocannabivarin (tetra-hydro-ka-nab-a-varin), is a semi intoxicating cannabinoid, and comes from cannabigerovarin acid (CBGVA), which is one of the two original minor cannabinoids. At this point it is THCVA, and we now know what happens to the "A" acid form when exposed to heat and/or light.[50]

THCV is found in very low concentrations in cannabis flowers, although breeders are working on making this minor cannabinoid more available.

Potential beneficial effects of THCV

- Inflammation
- Obesity
- Diabetes
- Neuroprotection
- Appetite Suppression

** There wasn't any sound research to warrant a slide on the negatives of THCV.**

---

[49]Brierley D. I., Samuels J., Duncan M., Whalley B. J., Williams C. M. (2017). A Cannabigerol-Rich Cannabis Sativa Extract, Devoid of Δ9-tetrahydrocannabinol, Elicits Hyperphagia in Rats. Behav. Pharmacol. 28, 280–284. 10.1097/fbp.0000000000000285\

[50]https://www.ncbi.nlm.nih.gov/pmc/articles/PMC8669157/

Delta 8 or D8 stands for Delta-8 tetrahydrocannabinol (tetra-hydro-ka-nab-a-nall), is intoxicating, and is a really close relative of D9 THC. The buzz can mimic that of THC, but on a more mellow level.[51]

Delta 8 is only found naturally in really, really low concentrations, so the majority of it is synthetically produced from a chemical conversion of CBD, usually from hemp.[52] My concern with this is that you really have to question the methods of those producing this chemically made cannabinoid, as it is mostly unregulated. The Farm Bill of 2018 gave them the loophole to sell it just about anywhere, but some states have required D8 to only be sold under their state-sanctioned medical marijuana programs. In my opinion, I believe this is the right call, as the state-required testing protocols are very much needed to keep these producers honest, and the product clean.

Potential beneficial effects of Delta 8

| Chronic Pain | Anxiety | Sleep Issues |

Potential negative effects of Delta 8

| Dry Mouth | Paranoia | Red Eyes |

| Increased Hunger | Sleep Issues |

A few years back, I visited a licensed processor in Oklahoma to see how they were manufacturing Delta 8, as it was very new to the cannabis industry. The last leg of the tour put us in the kitchen where their D8 gummies were being laid out prior to packaging. The chef offered us a sample of the gummies stating that they were 10 mg each. At the time, the extent of my knowledge was that D8 felt like a 1:1 in that it was a lower-key high. But knowing that I don't do well with edibles, and that I am rarely high in public, I bit the small candy in half and tossed the other half when no one was looking (stoners still judge).

---

[51]*https://www.ncbi.nlm.nih.gov/pmc/articles/PMC8669157/*
[52]*https://health.clevelandclinic.org/what-is-delta-8/*

Our tour wrapped up and we all headed out to lunch. I'm about halfway through my sandwich, and I realize that I am stoned out of my gourd! I did my best to maintain my composure throughout the rest of the meal but was thankful when the cold air in the parking lot hit my face. We returned to the facility, and once I was able to get my boss alone, I asked, "Are you high? I'm so high right now. I don't understand it. I only ate half!" The woman replied with, "I thought it was just me! What in the hell were in those things?" Not being as passive as I was, she flat-out asked the chef if he was absolutely sure they were only 10 mgs. And then the room began to chuckle at our expense.

"Pretty sure, but we're still working on it. That's the fun of R&D, isn't it? Ha-ha. You should've seen Jason when we slipped him 500 mgs. Hee-hee. Smacked his head pretty good on a coffee table. Ha-ha. Show them the scar Jason. Ha-ha." I was beyond livid that we had been roofied, and no longer saw them as professionals, but knuckle-dragging snails and puppy dog tails.

Usually I only have to stick my hand in the fire once to know that it will burn me, so I chalked this up as a teaching moment about the chemical conversions of synthetic cannabinoids.

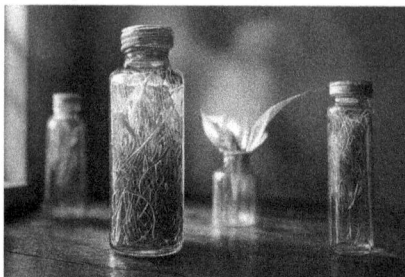

CHEMOTYPES, PHENOTYPES & GENOTYPES ... OH MY!

I have to mention the distinction between these three terms, so as not to upset my plant science peeps, and also to lay the groundwork for our collective hopes in changing the way we identify marijuana. You will find that I defer to a few people in this book who are experts in the fields that I still cannot confidently grasp enough to teach. Chemotypes, phenotypes, and genotypes, are a few such categories, and Josh Ferla is one such expert.

———

It was during the hazy, marijuana-filled summer days of the '80s in California's redwood-engulfed bay area that Josh found his natural affinity for plants. His fascination with the appearances, the smells, and the other characteristics of the cannabis plant turned Josh into a second-generation cannabis grower. Reagan years be damned, he experimented with friends and family, trying different cultivation methods and techniques. Once out on his own, he dove into the science of indoor cultivation and the chemistry of cannabis cultivation to dial in his craft.

After a few years of fine tuning his talent by working on cannabis farms and in dispensaries, Josh got into commercial-scale farming at the legendary Lost Coast of Humboldt County, 3,000 ft. above the cloud line. This is where he learned the art of organic, sustainable farming and responsible agricultural practices. Over the next few years, he grew his network of likeminded individuals that wanted integrity in their growing processes, both here in the U.S. and across the pond as well. Today, Mr. Ferla's state-of-the-art cannabis cultivation facilities that meet the highest of standards, and I can personally attest to the love he has for his compost and the seriousness of its role in growing clean, healthy cannabis.

Now, according to Josh, "Genotypes are the DNA of a particular cannabis plant. Its genetic gene pool if you will. Now, there will be different physical traits, phenotypes (fee-no-type), that show up after planting once it has been exposed to the environment (temps, humidity, indoor or outdoor stressors).

These physical traits can range from the very subtle to the not-so-subtle differences in plant structure, color, growth pattern, or vigor. Kind of like you and your maternal siblings can look similar but different from each other, even though you

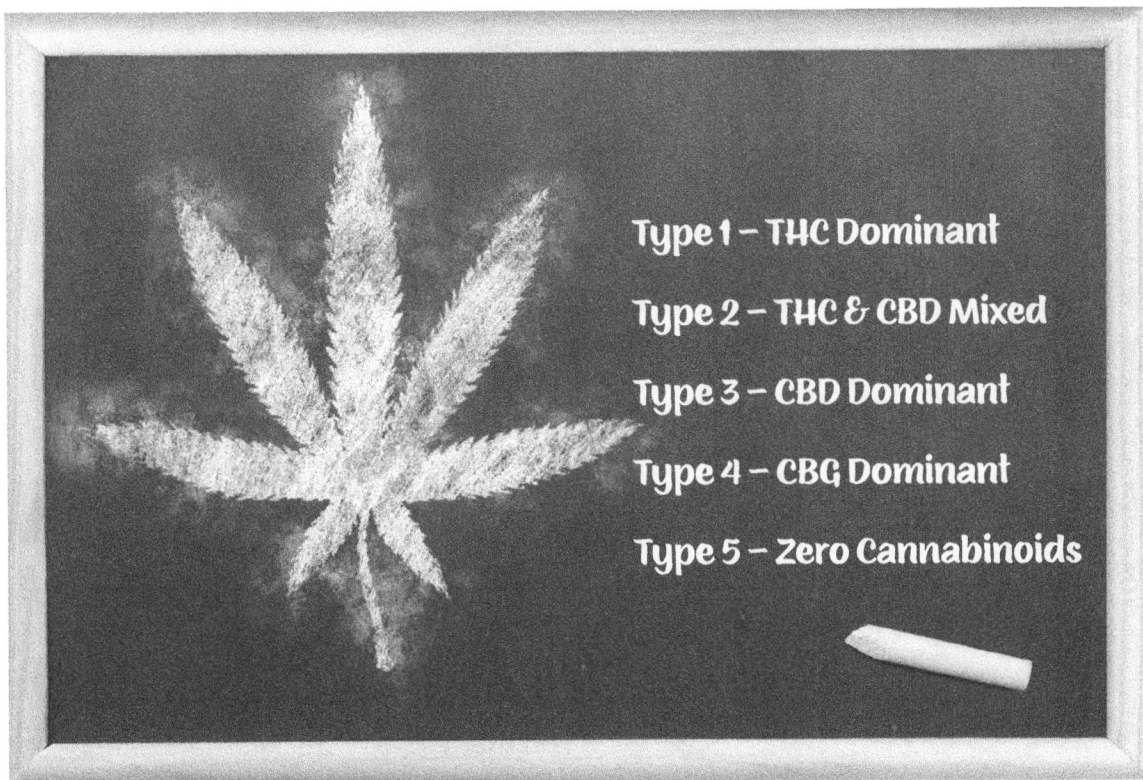

Type 1 – THC Dominant

Type 2 – THC & CBD Mixed

Type 3 – CBD Dominant

Type 4 – CBG Dominant

Type 5 – Zero Cannabinoids

share the same genotype—or genetic pool of material—and have been exposed to the same environment. Some of us tan better or burn easier than our siblings, have freckles etc."

Chemotypes, by definition, "... are often defined by the most abundant chemical profile produced by that individual and the concept has been useful in work done by chemical ecologists and natural product chemists."[53]

Josh explains even further with, "A chemotype is to plants as blue eyes, red hair, or inherited traits and health issues are to humans." Chemotypes characterize the most abundant chemical makeup, but also contain any potential deficiencies of the genetic material. So, even under perfect environmental conditions, you might get different physical attributes even though they come from the same gene pool. You see this in humans too; some families have twins and other strong resemblances to their children, other times kids with red hair are born to parents

---

[53]https://en.wikipedia.org/wiki/Chemotype

who have none. These are the expressions of the most abundant chemical make-up inherited from the genotype in that particular individual from the available gene pool, even including recessive genes.

"For instance, the Purple Punch cannabis strain also contains a fair amount of anthocyanins (water soluble pigments that can appear red, purple, or blue in cannabis flowers). However, some of the plant's physical traits expressed under certain environmental conditions (phenotypes), and their chemical makeup (chemotypes), did not acquire a large enough amount of anthocyanin chemicals from the gene pool (genotype) to produce these vibrant colors. This occurs even under the perfect environmental conditions, when other chemotypes might otherwise express these colors from the same exact genotype or genetic material."

Now I have done my due diligence (thanks to Mr. Ferla). But if this is an area that gets your wheels turning and your questions burning, I urge you to look further into it. Plant science can be pretty cool.[54]

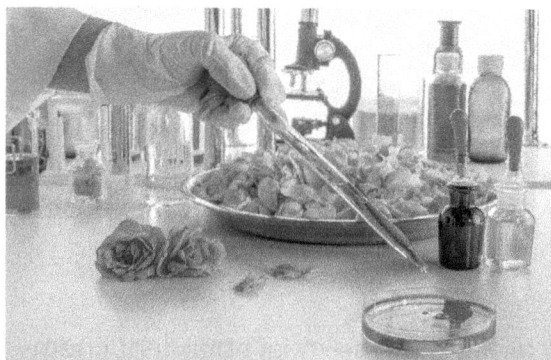

TERPENES

"Terps, terps, everywhere; in the stain on the wooden stair, in the shampoo in your hair,

In the magic of your bong, in the trichomes, thick and strong

Smell them here and taste them there; terps, terps, are everywhere...."[55]

Terpenes are defined as "... the largest and most diverse group of naturally occurring compounds that are mostly found in plants, but larger classes of terpenes such as sterols and squalene can be found in animals. They are responsible for the fragrance, taste, and pigment of plants ... The common plant sources of terpenes are tea, thyme, cannabis, Spanish sage, and citrus fruits (e.g., lemon, orange, mandarin)."[56]

---

[54]https://www.researchgate.net/publication/225323012_Time_course_of_cannabinoid_accumulation_and_chemotype_development_during_the_growth_of_Cannabis_sativa_L
[55]www.TheBigBookofTerps.com
[56]https://www.ncbi.nlm.nih.gov/pmc/articles/PMC7120914/

The more that I read about terpenes, the more impressed I am. Example, some plants can deploy an "indirect defense" where it actually puts out the call to the enemy of its enemies. For example, when white birch trees are under siege by moth caterpillars, the tree releases a blend of the terpenes ocimene and linalool. This terp blend attracts several species of birds that attack and feed on the caterpillars.[57]

Nature is so smart!

So, what can terpenes do for humans? The saying goes, "your nose knows." If your snout finds a certain aroma welcoming or is disgusted by a scent, the theory is that it can be a clue to what your body may actually need. Research has shown this to be particularly helpful in mood or anxiety disorders.[58]

———

Let's take a look at the most popular terpenes that can be found in cannabis.

Beta Caryophyllene (beta-carry-o-file-lean)
Is Beta Caryophyllene—or BCP for short—a cannabinoid? Or is it a terpene? It actually is both! BCP is often categorized as a cannabinoid, not a terpene, because it binds to CB2 cannabinoid receptors. That being said, it also has the ability to dampen the effects of THC when taken together. BCP is also found in abundance in several legal herbs and spices such as cinnamon, basil, pepper, coriander, chestnut, sage, lavender, oregano, and rosemary, among others. It is even an FDA-approved food additive, and for this reason, some sources label BCP the "first dietary cannabinoid."[59]

Studies are showing that BCP could potentially curb addiction withdrawals, assist with wound healing, and even be applied as a tumor suppressant.[60]

FLAVOR/AROMA
- Clove
- Dry
- Spicy
- Woody

HEALTH EFFECT
- Antimicrobial
- Anti-Inflammatory
- Neuroproductive

VAPORIZE AT:
130°C   266°K

[57]https://pubmed.ncbi.nlm.nih.gov/18665271/
[58]https://pubmed.ncbi.nlm.nih.gov/31481004/
[60]https://balancedbranches.com/research/beta-caryophyllene/

Delta-3-Carene (car-een)

Delta-3-Carene can smell like a sweet mix of pine, citrus, and wood, and can be found in pine and cedar trees, as well as rosemary. It is used as an insect repellent and in the cosmetic industry for perfumes.

Research is showing that this terpene can help with repairing damaged bones and fending off inflammation. Delta-3-Carene is unique due to its ability to draw out liquids. This makes it a good candidate to be used as an antihistamine, or for any other issue that may need fluids whisked away. But alas, this is a double-edged sword, as this little guy is mostly likely the culprit for the dry eyes and cottonmouth cannabis smoker's combat.[61]

FLAVOR/AROMA
- Pine
- Rosemary
- Cypress

HEALTH EFFECT
- Anti-Inflammatory
- Bone Stimulant

VAPORIZE AT:
- 171°C
- 340°K

Humulene (hum-a-leen)

What do beer and cannabis have in common? Hops! To be more specific, the terpene humulene, which smells of herbal spice and that classic peppery, hoppy bite. It can also be naturally found in cloves, sage, ginger, black pepper, and spearmint.

Humulene has strong anti-inflammatory properties and is still used today in Chinese medicine as an appetite suppressant.[62]

FLAVOR/AROMA
- Bitter
- Floral
- Peppery
- Woody

HEALTH EFFECT
- Antibacterial
- Anti-Inflammatory

VAPORIZE AT:
- 106°C
- 222°K

[61]https://onlinelibrary.wiley.com/doi/abs/10.1002/ptr.2247
[62]https://pubmed.ncbi.nlm.nih.gov/17559833/

Limonene (lem-in-neen)

Limonene is one of the most common terpenes out there. You can find this lemony scent in everything from your body lotion to your cleaning supplies. It can also be used as a "green" solvent in itself. So please keep this in mind if you are into concentrates with "terp sauce," and are considering cranking up the heat on your rig.

On the medical side of things, limonene has been studied for its anti-inflammatory, anticancer, antiviral, and gut-protecting effects. When consumed via cannabis, the effects can be uplifting and used as a mood stabilizer.[63] It is also showing promise because "d-Limonene has also been used as a sorption promoter or accelerant for improving transdermal drug delivery and works by penetrating the skin to reversibly decrease barrier resistance." So, if the next cannabis topical you buy has limonene in the ingredients, you just might be getting more bang for your buck.[64]

FLAVOR/AROMA
- Citrusy
- Sweet

HEALTH EFFECT
- Antibacterial
- Mood Elevation
- Stress Relief

VAPORIZE AT:

176°C   349°K

Linalool (lin-a-looool)

Would you agree that lavender is soothing and/or calming? What is giving off those effects is my favorite terpene, linalool, which can also be found in lavender, sage, rosemary, lemon balm, and bergamot.

This popular floral scent has been researched for uses as a natural aid for sleep issues, and as a calming agent for anxiety without the side effects of sedation, dependance, tolerance, or withdrawal symptoms.[65]

FLAVOR/AROMA
- Floral
- Rose
- Woody

HEALTH EFFECT
- Antianxiety
- Sedative

VAPORIZE AT:

199°C   390°K

---

[63]https://pubmed.ncbi.nlm.nih.gov/18665271/
[64]https://pubmed.ncbi.nlm.nih.gov/31481004/
[60]https://balancedbranches.com/research/beta-caryophyllene/
[65]https://www.ncbi.nlm.nih.gov/pmc/articles/PMC6007527/

Myrcene (mer-seen)

Myrcene is one of the most abundant, attractive-smelling terpenes found in cannabis. It can also be found in the oils of plants like hops, lemongrass, and citrus fruits.

FLAVOR/AROMA
- Citrusy
- Sweet

HEALTH EFFECT
- Antibacterial
- Mood Elevation
- Stress Relief

VAPORIZE AT:

176°C   349°K

In addition to the enticing smell of myrcene, it may aid other cannabinoids and terpenes in busting through the blood-brain barrier for better bio-availability. Cannabis strains that have over 0.5% myrcene are more likely to deliver the "couchlock" effects, and therefore would be known to the general public as an "indica." In turn, those with less than 0.5% would be leaning toward the giddy-up "sativa" end of the spectrum.

Current research reports that some of the biological activities include sedation, antidiabetic, antioxidant, anti-inflammatory, antibacterial, and possible anti-cancer effects.

According to the National Library of Medicine, there seems to be a disagreement on whether myrcene, as a food additive, is safe or is a tumor-causing carcinogen. "The uncertainty of the safety of myrcene stems from studies conducted by the National Toxicology Program, USA (NTP) which has shown an increased incidence of kidney and liver neoplasms in rodents. In 2018, the FDA took regulatory action to no longer permit the use of β-myrcene as a food additive based on legal action taken against the FDA under the Delaney Clause. (A federal health statute which prohibits FDA approval of any food additive which caused cancer in humans or animals.) Importantly, the FDA confirmed that there was no safety concern for β-myrcene to public health under the conditions of its intended use. Several other regulatory and scientific expert bodies have since argued that β-myrcene is safe under conditions of intended use as a flavouring substance and it must be noted that countless permitted food products continue to naturally contain significant levels of β- myrcene."[66]

So again, dabbers, you may want to back off the hellfire heat when inhaling terpenes in high concentrations. There is still so much that we don't know, and it is better to proceed with caution.

---

[66]https://www.ncbi.nlm.nih.gov/pmc/articles/PMC8326332/

Alpha & Beta Pinene (pine-een)

Pinene is nature's king of the terpenes, and they can also be found in basil, dill, orange peels and yep, you guessed it—pine needles. There are two, the alpha and the beta, and they both come with their own unique attributes.

Research is looking into this rockstar for its anti-inflammatory and anti-anxiety potential, plus its influence as a bronchodilator. Yes, the inhalation of this terpene will actually help open up your lungs! Studies have also reported that they may have the potential to reduce the number of lung cancer nodules, prevent gastric lesions, and show anticancer and antimicrobial promise.[67][68]

α-Pinene

FLAVOR/AROMA

- Cool
- Fresh
- Turpentine
- Herbal
- Piney

HEALTH EFFECT

- Alertness
- Memory Retention

VAPORIZE AT:

156°C   313°K

β-Pinene

FLAVOR/AROMA

- Piney
- Spicy
- Woody
- Green Hay

HEALTH EFFECT

- Anti-Inflammatory
- Bronchodilator

VAPORIZE AT:

156°C   313°K

[67] https://www.ncbi.nlm.nih.gov/pmc/articles/PMC6920849/
[68] https://www.ncbi.nlm.nih.gov/pmc/articles/PMC4329611/

FLAVONOIDS

Flavonols	Flavanols	Flavones	Anthocyanidins	Isoflavones	Flavanones
Examples	**Examples**	**Examples**	**Examples**	**Examples**	**Examples**
Myricetin, Kaempferol, Quercetin	EGCG, Epi-gallocatechin, Epicatechin, Catechin	Apigenin, Luteolin	Pelargonidin, Malvidin, Cyanidin	Daidzein, Genistein	Naringen-in, Hesperetin
Dietary Sources	**Dietary Sources**	**Dietary Sources**	**Dietary Sources**	**Dietary Sources**	**Dietary Sources**
Broccoli, Onions	Chocolate, Wine, Green Tea	Parsley, Celery	Berry Fruits, Red Wine	Soy, Soy Products	Citrus Fruits, Tomatos

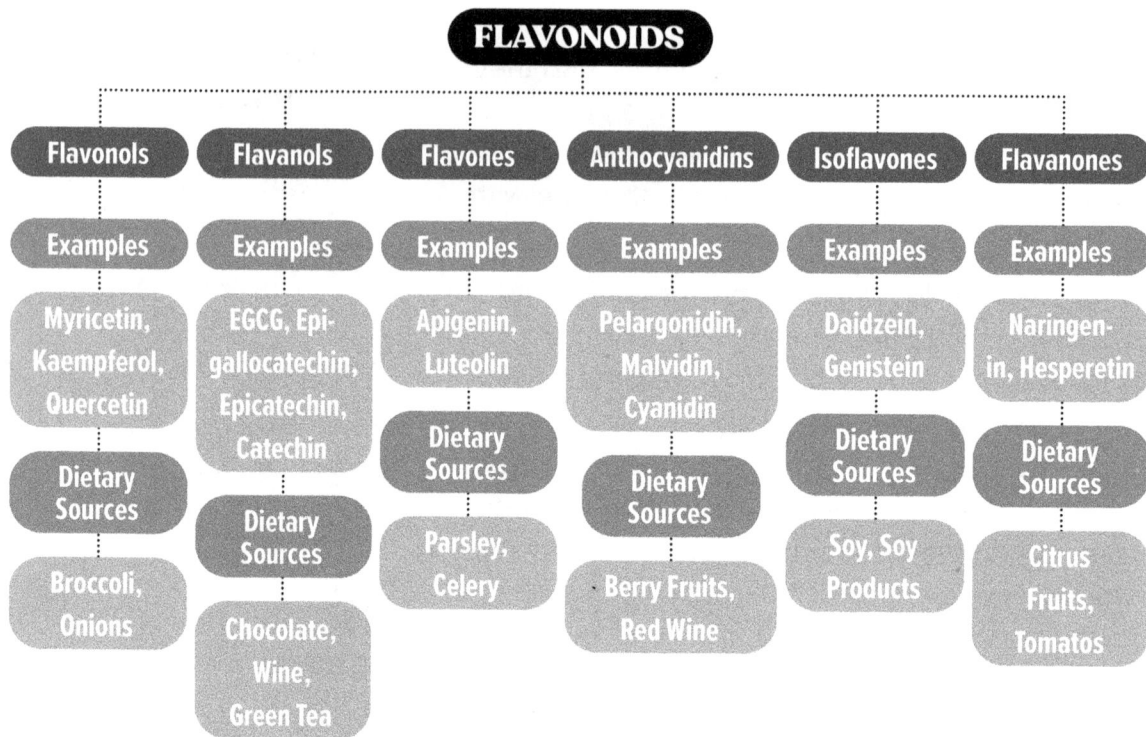

Even though terpenes are getting all the attention these days, we cannot forget the mighty flavonoid!

The National Library of Medicine reports that "Currently there are about 6000 flavonoids that contribute to the colourful pigments of fruits, herbs, vegetables and medicinal plants."

So, flavonoids have nothing to do with flavor (thanks, science, for making it confusing), but are actually in charge of the color of plants. Those amazing fall colors that we all love so much are brought to us by the flavonoid anthocyanins. When the cooler air comes to town, the chlorophyll begins to break down and allows for these colors to shine through.

In fruits they attract pollinators and therefore help with seed and spore germination and the growth and development of said seedlings. Flavonoids also play a part in toughening up for frosts, freezing tolerance, and resistance to drought.

Why is this important to the cannabis consumer? Because flavonoids also have medicinal properties such as anti-inflammatory, anti-mutagenic, and anti-carcinogenic superpowers.[69]

---

[69]https://www.ncbi.nlm.nih.gov/pmc/articles/PMC5465813/

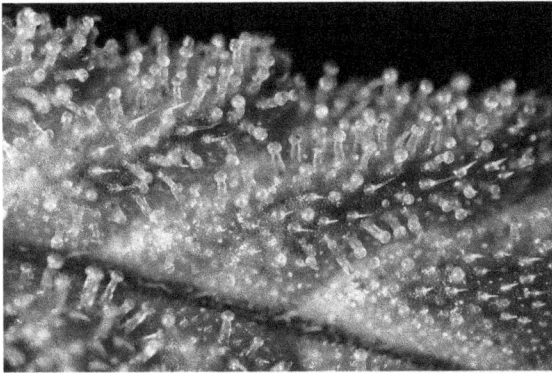

PLANT ANATOMY

And where are all of these amazing plant attributes housed, you may ask? Why, they are stored in the totally tubular oddities you see in the picture on the left called trichomes (try-combs), also known as the "frost" located on the outside of the plant.

Per Chapter 4 of the amazingly named paper, "The Botanical Dance of Death: Programmed Cell Death in Plants" we learn that "Trichomes are shoot epidermal hairs, found on the majority of plants, and are composed of either single or several cells (Esau, 1977). They play various protective roles, such as being a mechanical barrier to insect herbivores, filtering UV light and reducing respiration (Fordyce and Agrawal, 2001; Karabourniotis et al., 1992; Levin, 1973; Ripley et al., 1999; Van Dam and Hare, 1998)."[70]

So, one reason the sticky icky is sticky is to deter some pests from invading and setting up shop.

Landraces

A landrace strain is a pure cannabis plant that is exactly how and where God put it. This term is used to indicate the purity of its genetics, therefore meaning it has never been sliced, diced, or bastardized. "Sativa" landraces are originally from hot climates such as Africa, Jamaica, and South America. "Indica" landraces, on the other hand, are from cooler climates like the Afghan Mountains. A few famous landrace strains are Lambs Bread, Hindu Kush, Durban Poison, and Panama Red.

We have heard many growers throw around the term "landrace" when marketing their offerings. But are there truly any real landrace strains left in this labradoodle world? Some say yes and some say no. Just about everything on the dispensary shelves is a hybrid of some sort. So, there are those that spend their days "hunting" the four corners of our planet for the genotypes and phenotypes of moons gone by to build cannabis genetic bases in hopes of creating a baseline. Enter David Watson stage left....

---

[70]https://www.sciencedirect.com/science/article/abs/pii/B9780123858511000044

In the world of marijuana maestros, the co-founder of HortaPharm, David Watson, is a deity among men. He has collected the world's most extensive library of cannabis seeds known to man.[71]

As someone who is a lifetime member of the Seed Savers Exchange in the United States, it's safe to say that the guy really digs his seeds. And the potential for different medical applications, depending on the genetics, turned David's attention towards collecting cannabis seeds. In his travels during this quest, he had noticed that the worldwide attempts to wipe this plant out were putting more than a dent into the upper crust of the plant's genetic gene pool. So, with all possible speed Mr. Watson traveled to the far corners of the earth collecting what he could.

In 1994 he applied to the Dutch Ministry of Health for a license to grow cannabis, and in 1997 he and his business partner Robert Clarke became the first legal cannabis grow operation for pharmaceutical research.

When interviewed by Bill Breen in 2004, he was asked what exactly he was looking for in a cannabis plant. David had said, "I want varieties that have unusual characteristics in their growth or flowering period, or new and unusual sources of cannabinoids." And when he was asked why, he replied in a true salt of the earth fashion with "We were really interested in bringing cannabis back into mainstream medicine."[72]

The partners began HortaPharm, and with a proprietary process they became the planet's first breeder to develop homozygote cannabis called "selfing." This technique, in which both sets of chromosomes are identical, allows for the mass production of the cannabis plant with the same cannabinoid profile every time. This is huge! Because this is exactly what is needed if we are to turn botanicals into standard medications.

---

[71] https://www.accesswire.com/473598/Industry-Pioneer-David-Watson-Joins-United-Cannabis-Corp-Advisory-Board
[72] https://www.fastcompany.com/48172/dr-dopes-connection

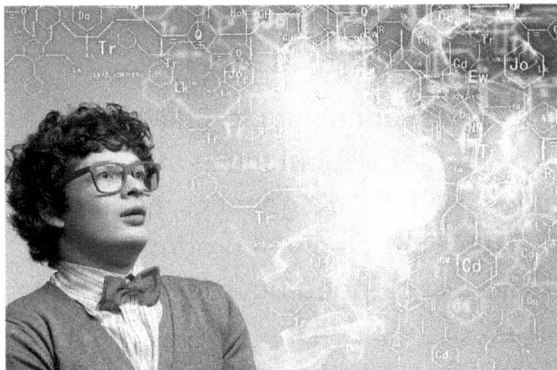

Indica, Sativa and Hybrids

We have all heard these terms before. Indica is supposed to give sedative effects of being "in-da-couch." Sativas are labeled as giving the opposite effects, offering the giddy-up that some of us lack. And then there is the hybrid, which claims to be a mix of both. To say that a flower "leans" one way or the other is again said to dictate if the product will be more sedative or energizing.

Sorry guys, but these terms are frankly misleading. Sativa and indica can be used when describing the physical attributes of how the plant grows and looks to the naked eye. But these terms have little to do with what is actually in the plant, chemically speaking.

I have spoken to many inquirers on the subject, and they are amazed when I tell them that THC was only a portion of the story when it came to their beloved "Sativas." I explained that it was the terpenes, such as pinene or limonene, that gave them the uplifting feeling they craved with their high.

> While on the subject of what's in a name, I'm going to push you a bit farther. Do not put too much stock into a strain's name. You could take three separate grams of Purple Punch, from three different locations, and the odds are that they would all have different profiles. By profiles, I mean the concentration of different cannabinoid and terpene amounts from the test results. Hell, I've named strains before myself. I was presented with a cross of Granddaddy Purple and a Durban Poison and asked what it was called for proper entry into the system. The response I got was a shoulder shrug and "what should we call it?" So, I deemed it Granddaddy Durban, and so it was.

1:1 Ratios

Now I have only run across a few people that have very high tolerances for THC, but when they combine it with CBD, it puts them in a completely different frame of mind. One fella I know has smoked heavy amounts of marijuana on every single continent, yet when we shared a bowl of Cannatonic #4 (high CBD) with Apollo 13 bubble hash (high THC) sprinkled on top, he was floored! The vast majority of us will not feel this type of effect, but this is a good example of how different mixtures of cannabinoids can have different effects on each of us.

Most of us don't usually consider mixing the two cannabinoids, unless you are like me that adores a natural 1:1 ratio for pain relief without much of a high. By "natural," I mean both THC and CBD are a part of the plant's genetics, and have close to even amounts of each cannabinoid. There are plenty of products out there that are sold as a 1:1, but most of them are just stripped-down THC distillate mixed with CBD isolate. This splicing and dicing of the cannabis plant gives different results than when you keep as much of the plant together as possible.

Unfortunately, you'll be hard pressed to find true 1:1 flower in retail shops. When I approach growers about this their answers are all the same. "It doesn't sell." Or "It doesn't yield enough to make it worth my time". Ugh. I believe that if retailers and patients alike were educated on the benefits of this ratio, the shops would sell it in abundance. But instead, we are stuck with mixing THC strains with hemp flower for the CBD.

SOME WELL-KNOWN 1:1 STRAINS INCLUDE:

- Harlequin
- AC/DC
- Startonic
- Pennywise
- Girl Power
- Milk & Cookies

I am going to jump ahead here briefly to help make sure that the following section makes a little more sense. Before we get into the different ways someone can use cannabis, I want you to understand that the amount of product that gets into your system depends not on just the volume you take, but on how you take it. This is known as bioavailability, and is defined as, "When a substance such as a medicine or supplement enters your system, the portion of the total substance introduces which can effectively create a response determines that substance's bioavailability. The bioavailability of a substance can fluctuate, depending on the route of administration.

—

"Intravenous administration, or a direct line into the bloodstream, is typically considered 100% bioavailability, as all of the substance will reach target cells. In oral administration routes, AKA when you take a pill, the amount of medicine or supplement you receive depends on many factors, including your diet and your personal metabolism."[73]

———

That being said, how much and how fast you are affected has almost every-thing to do with how you choose to take your cannabis. Notice that I said "al-most?" That is because genetics and tolerance will also have their say in how and when your weed kicks in as well.

And then there is the decarboxylation (dee-car-box-a-lay-shun) we were talking about when changing acid forms (THCA + heat = THC). Cannabinoids all have different boiling points, and unless you want to scorch your stash to ash, you should know how hot is too hot.

248°F	THCA & CBG
266°F	CBDA
283°F	CBCA

311°F	Delta 9 THC
329°F	CBD
347°F	Delta 8 THC

365°F	CBN
393°F	CBE
428°F	THCV & CBD

- Ex: You want to make cannabis cookies with some shake you bought at your local pot shop. You know you have to change the THCA to THC by decarbing the plant matter first, but if you pop it in the oven at 400 degrees you will be cooking off all of the THC that was intended for your tagalongs.[74]

---

[73]https://biologydictionary.net/bioavailability/
[74]https://www.veriheal.com/blog/cannabinoid-boiling-points-a-guide-to-optimal-vaporizer-temperatures/

THE FIVE METHODS OF INTAKE

Now we can get into the top five most common ways to partake. These are inhaling, ingesting, sublingually, topical application, and bringing up the rear—rectally.

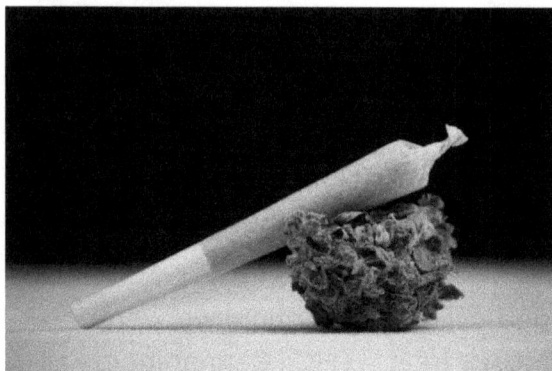

Inhaling:
Joints vs. Vaporizing vs. Cartridges

The quickest route, outside of sticking a needle in your arm (nobody should ever, ever do this), is to inhale. You can roll a joint or a blunt. You can pack a bowl, fire up a bong, or use a dry herb vaporizer. The dried flower of the cannabis plant (buds, nugs or the thousand other names to call it) is still the most popular method of consumption.[75]

Once you roll it up and set a flame to it, you are now not only inhaling the herb, but also the paper and the carcinogens common with the whole smoking process. When you use a bong or bowl (I recommend glass), you are getting the herb and the carcinogens. But if you choose to use a dry herb vaporizer you are getting nothing but the plant with each hit. This is due to the process of vaporization, where you are applying heat to the herb without actually burning the plant matter. After finishing what you put into the vape, you will not find ashes, as you would in a bowl or bong. What you will find is what looks like crispy, dry tobacco.

Studies have shown that the consumer can get up to 80% of the cannabinoids and terpenes (the good stuff) when vaporized, compared to the old school method where you are only getting up to 30% of the original goodness.[76]

I know, I know. Most of us old schoolers still prefer classic combustion to healthier alternatives. Maybe it's the draw into the lungs, maybe it's the release on exhale, or maybe the ceremonial preparation of rolling a joint or stuffing your

---

[75]https://flowhub.com/learn/top-selling-cannabis-products
[76]Medicinal Cannabis: In Vitro Validation of Vaporizers for the Smoke-Free Inhalation of Cannabis - PMC (nih.gov)

---

favorite bong. Regardless of our personal reasons, at least we have choices these days when it comes to how we smoke our cannabis.

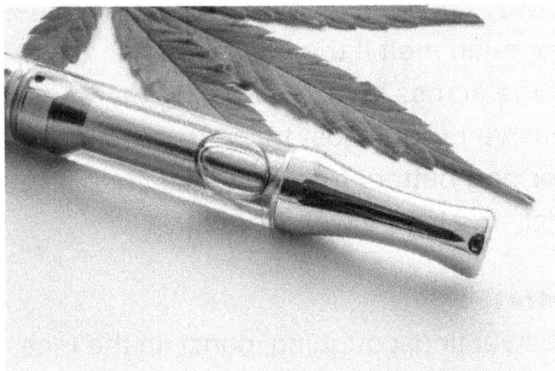

———

Things have become a bit more convenient for those who choose to inhale their marijuana with the invention of the cartridge. They are small, generally don't have a smell to them, and they seem to last forever. But hear me and heed me when I say that it is not the same as smoking flower.

Not even a little bit.

For starters, it isn't a flower. It is an end result of an extraction of the cannabis plant. It can be made from trim leaves or from the buds or from both. It is then processed by using solvents (we'll get into the different types later), and the end product is the highly concentrated oil product you see in your cartridges. Straight distillate carts are generally a very pale gold color, unless they are exposed to too much sunlight, in which case they will start to turn a darker color as the oil oxidizes. Resin and rosin carts, on the other hand, start out much darker, as there is more plant matter left behind in the end product.

Vaping and vaporizing use two completely different products. As mentioned above, vaporizing is using the dried flower, while vaping is using concentrated cannabis. Vaping, whether it's cannabis or nicotine, has been a very real health concern for years. The illicit market, in true drug dealer fashion, has been making black market carts that have been repeatedly "stepped on," meaning that they take the original product and keep cutting the oil with Lord knows what to stretch their base product.

But there is a way for you to check to see if it's been severely diluted. Simply find the bubble in the oil and then flip your cart upside down. If the bubble races to the other end, it has been diluted. With uncut concentrates, the bubble will not move, or if it does, it will be extremely slow about it. This of course is not foolproof, just a little trick I picked up along the way.

Carts can come in a cylinder shape or in a pod shape. One is not better than the other, although they each use different batteries. It just comes down to a matter of preference.

Carts are notorious for malfunctioning. They can leak all over, clog up from the oil getting into the mouthpiece (yuck), or even melt if the battery temps are too hot. I have had more than one vaper come across my path whining that they clogged their tank or wasted a ton of expensive product just trying to get it in the damn thing. You can pick up any stick or pod battery from a smoke shop for cheap; try to get one with a temperature dial, and it'll be well worth it.

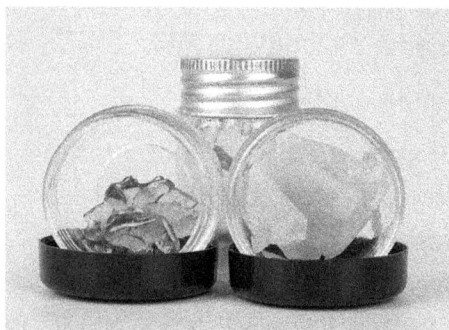

Concentrates

Ahh, the sweating, coughing, punch in the face of THC that entices those that are looking for the stronger effects of cannabis. I can see why some people can be concerned about the potency of some of today's cannabis products. Concentrates need to be respected, with cannabinoid percentages creeping in at over 90%.

Even though they are not my personal preference, I do believe that these concentrates, and their potency levels, do have their place in the world for cannabis medical patients. When a person is battling off-the-charts pain from chemo, or is trying to kick an opioid addiction, sometimes the only thing that will touch the pain is the one-two punch of concentrates. And when given proper direction, the patient can begin to wean themselves down to lower THC percentages over time, and therefore in theory will need less medication for their conditions.

There are several different ways to extract all of the goodies that a cannabis plant has to offer. Different methods will not only have an effect on the potency of the end product but can also have varying consistencies. My hope for you is that you'll be able to spot the extraction method based upon what it looks like on the shelf, and then not only be able to make confident guesses as to the general ballpark of the potency, but also how much of the original plant is still intact.

In the following section you will see the terms "plant matter" and "total cannabinoids" used quite a bit. Plant matter refers to the entire plant. Not only cannabinoids, terpenes, and flavonoids, but chlorophyll, lipids, waxes, and other compounds in the natural state of the plant. Total cannabinoids refer to the complete count of not only THC and CBD percentages, but also any cannabinoids detected that show up in testing, regardless of their low numbers.

———

Since concentrate knowledge is one part plant science and one part chemistry (neither one my strong suit), I have asked someone who knows these two subjects intimately to review and comment in the following section for accuracy and clarity.

Raven Ariola M.Sc. began his official cannabis career providing hands-on technical analysis and solutions to nearly every licensed cultivation and processing facility in Pennsylvania. It was in these medical cannabis testing labs, licensed grow facilities, and vertically integrated dispensaries that Raven saw the true results of what strong education can do for our rapidly growing industry.

He has received his degree in Medical Cannabis Sciences & Therapeutics from the University of Maryland School of Pharmacy, which is the nation's first graduate program studying cannabis science. He then served as the Director of Education for the Medical Cannabis Student Association. He is also responsible for the wildly popular podcast Plants Saved My Life, which offers the very personal experiences (mine included) that people have had with using plants as medicine.

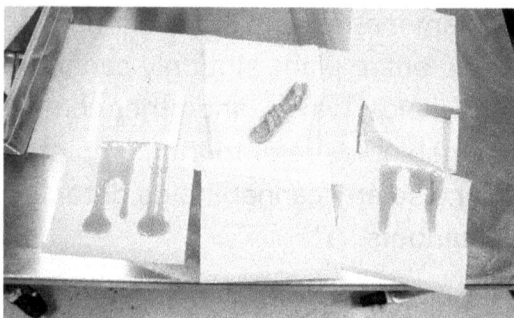

DIFFERENT EXTRACTION METHODS
Solvents vs. Solventless

Many solvents can be used when extracting cannabis for concentrates, but they can also be done without them. Using chemicals to pull out the desired plant compounds leads to some of the solvent being left behind. The product then needs to be run through a "purge" to clean up the product as much as possible. Most states have a list of "acceptable" levels of chemicals allowed in the end product, which can range from alcohols to gasses such as butane. Testing for these leftovers is crucial, especially for those that use concentrates as medicine. The very last thing a sick person needs is to intake these residuals at potentially toxic levels.

Even though some processors believe that concentrating the plant will "clean up" any contaminants, they are mistaken. In their attempts to concentrate the terpenes and cannabinoids, they are also concentrating any pesticides, heavy metals, and impurities as well.

But the purge is an unnecessary step when you don't use solvents to begin with. Pressure and heat can be used and will give you rosin in the end. Or you can use mesh bags to either add ice water, or without anything at all, to produce hash.

Some will argue that ice and water are not to be considered "solventless," as you are in fact using something to pull the goodies off of the plant. Others will go another way and say the CO_2 must be included as "solventless" because it is a natural product (even if it is converted from a gas to a liquid), like water and ice. It all comes down to who you ask.

It is these varying opinions that make the need for standardization crucial. When asking Raven this question, his educated opinion was "I'd define solventless as using NO solvent, including CO_2. Although water is 'the universal solvent,' it maintains the integrity of cannabinoids and terpenes. Anything using only heat and/or water is considered to be solventless."

Hashish

Hash is old, old school. In fact, it has been around for hundreds of years, and originated in places such as Morocco, Afghanistan, Nepal, Iran, and Lebanon.[77]

This concentrate is made by collecting and pressing the trichomes into a thick, tarry substance. It is then pressed into blocks or turned into oil. It is most commonly smoked or added to foods and teas.[78]

When speaking of hashish, one must give glory to Frenchy Cannoli. It has been said that he treated creating hash like raising a fine wine. He was relentless in his pursuit of obtaining and then aging this eras-old concentrate. I can think of no other person that respected this ancient way of concentrating cannabis more, and he was tireless in his teachings to spread the methods of yesteryears. If you are interested in the true art of hash making, I urge you to look into the education Frenchy has left behind for us.[79]

Ice Water/Bubble Hash

Modern hash is processed differently and is actually really hard to find in the retail shops. If I had to guess it would be because any leftover plant matter is being

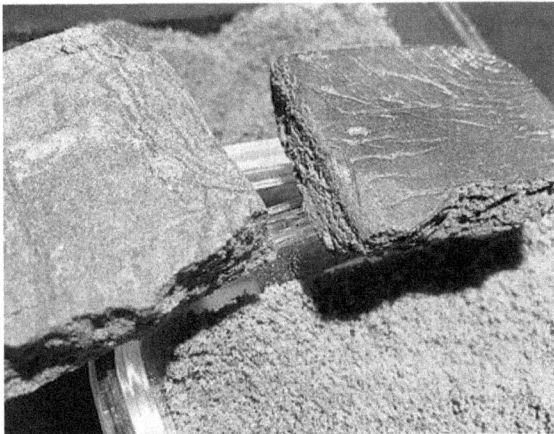

turned into higher THC percentage (and higher dollar worth) distillate, plus it is a total pain in the ass to make. The process is very hands-on and is more labor intensive than most processors are willing to do. Even though solventless is the most cost-efficient way to get started in extractions, the yield of only 5%-15% of weight is less than ideal for processors.

[77]https://druglibrary.org/MedicalMj/hash/history_of_hashish.htm
[78]https://www.drugs.com/illicit/hashish.html
[79]https://www.frenchydreamsofhashish.com/

Bubble hash was given its name due to the product actually bubbling when set on fire. It's made by using a series of mesh bags with varying-sized holes and simple ice water. The shimmying and shaking of the mesh bags will separate the partially frozen trichomes from the rest of the plant matter. One will also need a freeze dryer to rid the concentrate of excess moisture. The end product, once dry, will look crumbly and dark brown. This can be used as is, or further pressed into rosin.

This can also be done without the ice water, known as "dry sift," which is pretty much just kief, as the process is just knocking off the cannabinoid and terpene-filled trichomes.

Consumers have reported that by going this route the end product has less "flavor," which is probably due to beating up the trichomes during the extraction process. You can expect the potency to range from 55% to 65% total cannabinoids.

Pressure and Heat

The simple actions of applying the right temperature and then pressing the living hell out of a bud will give you a solventless concentrate called rosin. This is sometimes referred to as "squishing," and the end result is a dark and thick syrupy product. The color not only comes from the whole plant properties, but also from burnt plant matter, which makes rosin a partial decarbed product.

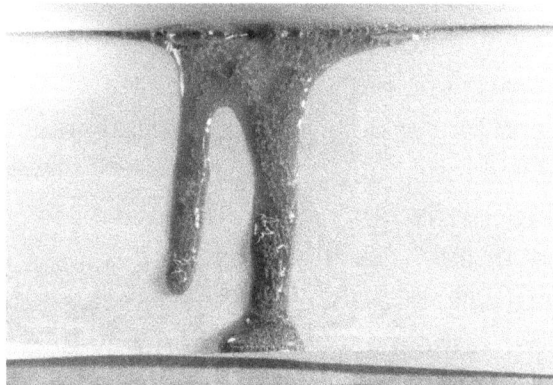

Just about anyone who is into concentrates has tried to produce rosin by putting a bud between two pieces of wax paper and using a hair straightener in an attempt to squeeze out the concentrate. As these folks have learned—at the expense of a wasted nug or two—the process doesn't require a change to the method, but needs to be done on a much, much bigger scale with a much bigger hair straightener.

As with any high-heat extraction, the lesser terpenes and cannabinoids will be cooked off in the process, and therefore the potency numbers will be lower than some other methods. You can expect the end product strength to come in between 60%–80% total cannabinoids (depending on what you're working with). And if you are interested in the yields, it's typically about 10% of however much flower is used, according to Raven.

CO2 (Carbon Dioxide)

Carbon Dioxide, according to Britannica, is well known for its use as a refrigerant, in fire extinguishers, coal blasting, and promoting the growth of plants in greenhouses, among other things.[80]

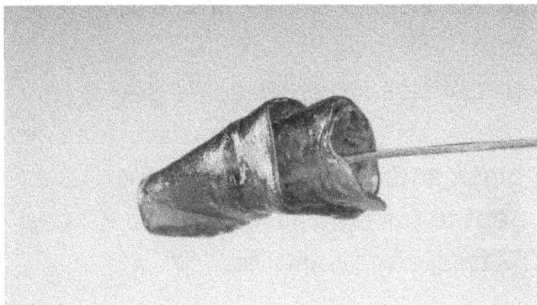

Now we can add cannabis extraction to this list.

Making concentrates using CO2 is done by turning this natural gas into a liquid and then applying it as a solvent. This method isn't as harsh on the plant and therefore leaves more of the original plant intact. But you will lose some of the minor terpenes, as they are usually the first to go in using the majority of extraction methods. When using CO2, you can have a more stable shelf life, and the product can last up to a year with minimal degradation if refrigerated to preserve the cannabinoids and terpenes. This is also assuming the concentrate is only exposed to minimal light and oxygen.[81]

The end product consistency is a lot like molasses in color and texture, and the potency can range from 60% to 80% total cannabinoids.[82]

BHO (Butane Hash Oil)

Using butane was once the most popular extraction method in retail, although I believe that distillate may be giving it a run for its money these days. In hearing

---

[80]https://www.britannica.com/science/carbon-dioxide
[81]https://www.extractz.com/what-is-co2-extraction
[82]https://medium.com/@Z_Lucie/cannabis-extractions-the-complete-guide-151edb382d65

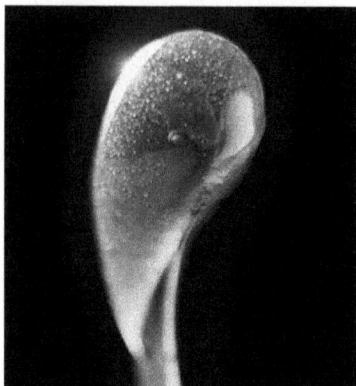

of homemade extractions, and the garages they have leveled over the years, you can almost guarantee that it was due to the reckless use of butane and their attempts to purge.

———

After the butane, propane, or other "anes" (hydrocarbons) have been run through the plant matter, "you are then left with roughly 95% cannabis oil and 5% propane or butane residual solvents in your collection pot. At this point it still needs the 72-hour purge."[83]

Different times and temps used during the purge will give you the different consistencies that you see in the shops. Some are shatter (glass-like), some are waxy and look like honeycombs, while others will look like apple sauce or whipped butter (badder, in retail speak). These physical consistencies play a role in what concentrate you may choose. Some prefer to "work with" badder for easy scooping, instead of shatter that breaks like glass and can fly everywhere. Butane extractions will still need to be decarbed by heat to turn the THCA into THC, and these can test out anywhere from 80% to 90% total cannabinoids.

Before the days of solvent restrictions, homogeneity, and "acceptable limits," extractionists were just learning the art of the purge. A lot of outbuildings burned down, and a lot of people consumed some pretty nasty concentrates, or "butane soup" as it is also known.

Yes, these guys also had to submit test results, and were often turned away with their pizza boxes filled with slabs of shatter with the warning to "do better," before trying to get in the door again. But these were the days when a fully stocked display case with questionable offerings was better than having only a handful of pricey stellar products. Concentrates are generally only purchased by the younger generation and therefore the bang for your buck is definitely top priority. Shady or ignorant, those were the times.

---

[83]https://terpenesandtesting.com/butane-extraction-101/

You could physically see who was buying the cheap "butane soup." Their skin was gray, eyes yellowed, and they were always cranky. Attempts to sway them toward cleaner concentrates were always met with an argument over pricing, and then the purchase of the same old crap.

Distillation

You can thank distillate for getting rid of the weedy taste in your edibles. Distillate was a game changer when it made its first appearance in the cannabis market. It pushed cartridges into the daylight, it was an easier, more consistent product to infuse edibles with, and is generally free of everything except the desired THC.

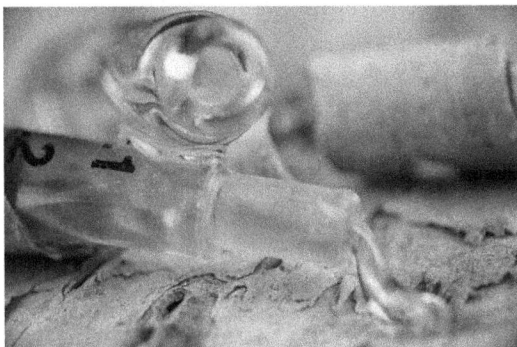

Think along the lines of a gin mill south of the Mason-Dixon. Everything is broken down to the compound level, then temperature is used to cook off everything but the THC (sometimes CBD). More often than not, cannabis processors will take the plant and turn it into a butane extraction before using the distillate process to refine it even further. Distillate is considered to be a single, completely decarbed compound product—unless terpenes are reintroduced—and can test out in the mid to high 90% range.

Tip: If your distillate is being difficult in that you cannot seem to get it out of the syringe, you can either rub it between your hands or run it under warm water to get it to loosen up. When doing the latter, make sure you don't do it for too long. If the product gets too viscous, it will all come dripping out once you have removed the cap.

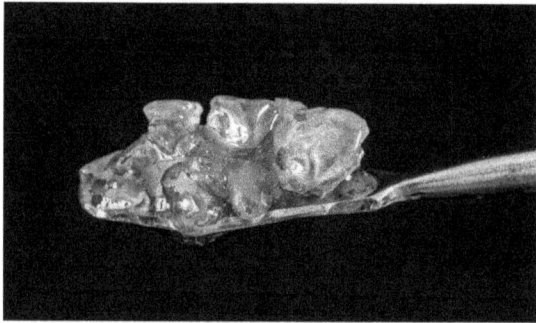

THCA Diamonds and Sauce

These "diamonds," sometimes called "sand," are just about as close as you can get to pure THCA (96%–99.9%), although you may find very small amounts of other cannabinoids and terpenes in the end product (1%–4%). THCA diamonds are considered the most potent single cannabinoid extract option currently available.

———

So how can you tell how potent your diamonds will be just by looking at them? The diamonds highest in THC will be a stark snow white. If there are some terpenes and/or cannabinoids that hang around, the product will have an amber or yellowish hue.[84] These "leftovers" are not a bad thing. If I was shopping for diamonds, I would actually choose the less pristine option for the added terpenes and cannabinoids.

But the visual purity of the diamonds will be lost when combined with "sauce," which is liquified terpenes mixed in for flavor and potential effects. Also, please remember my warning about inhaling terpenes in high concentrations with high heat once you get your purchase home.

———

Now I will leave the explanation of how these diamonds are made to Raven … "The process itself is actually pretty neat—technicians start with a processed extract, then the crystals are 'grown' in mason jars using time and agitation when necessary. Remember the old science fairs where you'd scratch a glass, and salt would form? Same concept in crystal formation of THCA diamonds."

---

[84]*https://extraktlab.com/thca-diamonds/*

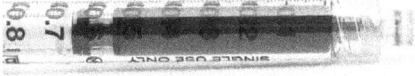

Alcohol

According to Johnsons Environmental Products, "Food grade alcohol" means ethyl alcohol that is safe for human consumption because of its purity (i.e., lack of additives). Period. Food grade alcohol goes by many names in the industry, including: food grade ethanol, nondenatured alcohol, grain alcohol, 190 proof grain, food grade EtOH, and Anhydrous Ethanol.[85]

———

As in any commercial production, people are always trying to cut corners to save a buck. Many cannabis processors will reach for the cheaper (and unacceptable) "denatured alcohol," which brings nasty carcinogens into the mix.

Now just because most of the above are considered "safe," does not mean that the extraction doesn't need to be purged. There is still a boatload of unwanted solvent after this extraction process, all of which must be flushed to meet any state sanctioned acceptable levels.

This method will give you the darkest color of all of the different extractions, as it holds onto the most plant matter, and will give you a whole plant extract that will generally test out between 50% to 75% total cannabinoids.

It is also the process most widely used for RSO (Rick Simpson Oil) or FECO (fully extracted cannabis oil). If you want to get technical, RSO is/was extracted with naphtha. "Humans commonly use petroleum naphtha as a solvent. It can be found in various cleaning agents where its low evaporation point comes in handy, and works as a dilution agent for paints, varnish, and asphalt. Dry-cleaning businesses also use naphtha in their operations."[86] Hence the reason for getting away from this solvent.

———

The "proposed" regimen for taking this extraction for the purposes of combating chemotherapy and cancer, is to take 90 grams in 60 days. This is a huge ask,

---

[85]https://enviroprod.com/blogs/news/what-is-food-grade-alcohol
[86]https://sciencing.com/naphtha-uses-7665916.html

especially for those brand-spanking-new to cannabis. Even with the beginning doses starting at a half of the size of a grain of rice, the struggle is real. Most will get a tolerance to this tarry substance rather quickly, but believe me when I tell you that the first two weeks will be a challenge.

I do have to mention that the RSO acronym is another frustrating bit of vernacular to some of us because it references the name of a "who" rather than "what" the product actually is. FECO (fully extracted cannabis oil) is the correct way to reference this type of product. I know. There are more than a few desired changes to the language used in this industry, but I promise it's only for a better understanding of the marijuana in our lives.

"Live" vs. "Cured" Concentrates

"Live" is when the plant is pulled out of the ground and is directly frozen at some pretty wicked cold temps to flash freeze all of the trichomes prior to extraction. This method will give you more of the original plant attributes and its flavors. "Cured" means that the plant was pulled and then dried before the extraction. And it should be taken into consideration that a cannabis plant can lose up to 75% of terpenes during the harvesting, drying, and curing process. This is also why you'll see "live" concentrates costing more in shops than the "cured" variety.

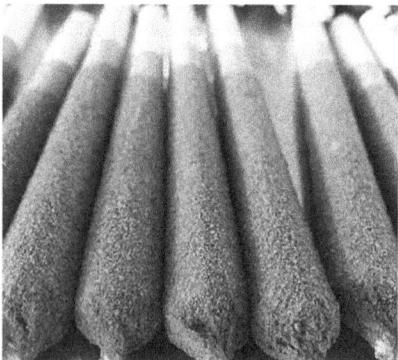

Two common questions often asked about concentrates are whether you can add them to your flower, and at what temperature you should smoke them at.

As anyone can tell just by looking at a dispensary menu, yes, you can in fact add concentrates to your flower, as infused joints are a big hit with consumers. But understand that adding any type of concentrate to your flower will increase the potency, and this should always be taken into consideration if you want to remain consistent with your dosages. It will also be a bit messier, as the resin will be thicker than if it was just flower alone.

Under this category you will find variations of "tarantula legs" and "moonrocks." The tarantula leg is a joint rolled in concentrate (usually hash oil unless specified otherwise) and then rolled again in kief or hash, giving it the appearance of a fuzzy spider leg.

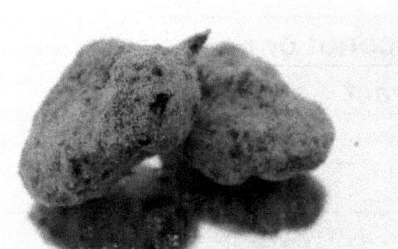

Moonrocks are the same concept without the paper. A bud is rolled in concentrate and then rolled again in hash or kief. Either of these will take your THC percentage rates from the mid-20s to the mid-60s.

As for the ideal temperature when smoking cannabis concentrates out of a rig (basically a bong for concentrates), it again comes down to who you ask. Some choose a hellfire temp to make sure all of the THCA is decarbed into THC smoke, wasting nothing. For those of us who have common sense, it doesn't have to be explained why inhaling a product at 700+ degrees is bad for your lungs. The other opinion is that "you have to waste it to taste it." Lower temperatures will allow for some of the more robust terpenes and cannabinoids to survive the trip to your lungs, but you may be leaving some of the non decarbed THCA behind.[87]

Note: If you have chosen to inhale your cannabis (either in the form of flower or concentrates), and you are a very new-to-cannabis user, I urge you to go responsibly slow. Take one hit. Just one. Give it some time to see how it makes you feel. Pay attention to both your physical and mental reactions. Then, if it didn't get you to where you wanted to be, hit it again. An important part of using cannabis as medicine is trial and error, and you have to be patient and pay attention if you truly want to get the most out of your medicine. Two drags off of a joint may be all you need, while others may need to smoke the whole thing. We are all different!

---

[87] https://keytocannabis.com/low-temp-dabs-vs-high-the-perfect-temperature-for-dab-potency-and-flavor/

ACRONYMS TO KNOW:

FECO	Fully Extracted Cannabis Oil
RSO	Rick Simpson Oil
MCT	Medium-Chain Triglycerides (from coconut or palm kernel oil)
HCFSE	High Cannabinoid Full Spectrum Extract
HTFSE	High Terpene Full Spectrum Extract
BHO	Butane Hash Oil
MIP	Marijuana Infused Product
PPM	Parts Per Million

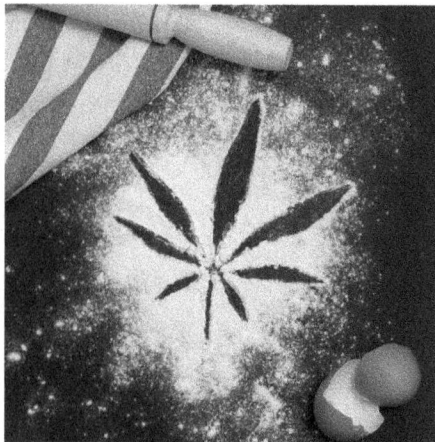

Edibles

Most people are shocked when I tell them that when they eat an edible, at best they are actually only getting up to 30% of the THC they just ate. When your cookie or gummy goes straight down the hatch, it is run through the gauntlet of our digestive system and loses its punch as it is being absorbed along the way. To top it off, THC (Delta-9) is completely changed at the chemical compound level once it hits the liver.[88]

Stay with me here folks.

We have a liver enzyme called P450, and according to the Mayo Clinic, "The human body uses cytochrome P450 enzymes to process medications. Because of inherited (genetic) traits that cause variations in these enzymes, medications may affect each person differently."[89]

[88]https://pubmed.ncbi.nlm.nih.gov/4729039/
[89]https://www.mayoclinic.org/tests-procedures/cyp450-test/about/pac-20393711

This enzyme can actually make our medications more or less potent, depending on the drug. Our nonintoxicating friend CBD is well known for blocking the potency of drugs metabolized by this enzyme.[90]

P450 is the magician that changes the THC that we started with into 11-Hydroxy THC, and therefore alters the effects. Many people report that eating something infused with THC and smoking THC result in very different highs. I have to agree, because no matter how many chances I give 11-Hydroxy THC, we just don't get along.

Ingesting cannabis can take anywhere from 30 minutes to a full two hours to kick in. This is when people tend to lose their patience and add more edibles into the mix, thinking that it's not working. Rookie mistake. Your metabolism, whether you took them on a full stomach, and/or your tolerances have everything to do with your projected launch time.

We have all heard the term "low and slow" when it comes to taking edibles, and I stress this point again for those of you in the cheap seats.

These little nuggets of extraction covered in sugar can last for hours on end, and if you hit the boxing ring too hard, too fast, well ... down goes Frazier. What also happens is that you are not any closer to figuring out what your milligram "sweet spot" really is. In the long run, you'll end up spending way more money on finding the right dose and product line.

—

Someone who works behind a cannabis counter long enough will eventually get to know the regular customers. There was a young man who was attending classes at the university up the road, and like clockwork he would come in every Thursday after school for his treasured flower. One day Jack cheerfully bounced into the med room and asked for 25 Rice Krispy treats for a skiing trip he was taking with his fraternity brothers. The wise old elder in me rose up, and warnings of how edibles are different came spilling out of my mouth; the 50 mg treat would pack a punch in a way that he was not accustomed to.

He humored me with a nod and then a request for the total, so I began to bag up the treats. I wished him luck and sent him on his way to tackle the mountain.

---

[90]*https://pubmed.ncbi.nlm.nih.gov/26651971/*

The following week, he returned to the counter via crutches. "Wasn't wrong, was I Jack?" I scolded. Bashfully he told me the backstory of how they ate the edibles about an hour before getting on the chairlift, and found that once up there they couldn't get down. They were so high that they just laid around at the lift drop off point for hours until they began to come down. Jack wasn't over his buzz as much as he thought he was before making the trip down the hill and misjudged the girth of a lone pine tree. He snapped his femur in two places and would need corrective surgery in the very near future. Still shaking my head at him, I sent him on his way with some flower to help with the pain.

Note: If you have chosen to eat your cannabis and are a very new-to-cannabis user, I'm still going to keep urging you to take it oh so slow. And by slow, I mean start with a product that has 5 mg pieces you can cut in half, take the 2.5 mgs and give it a full two hours before consuming any more. One of the differences between smoking and eating your weed is that even if you overdo it when smoking a joint, the buzz should pass in under two hours. But as mentioned above, if you consume too many milligrams in a sitting you could be saddled with an uncomfortable buzz for up to 8 hours.

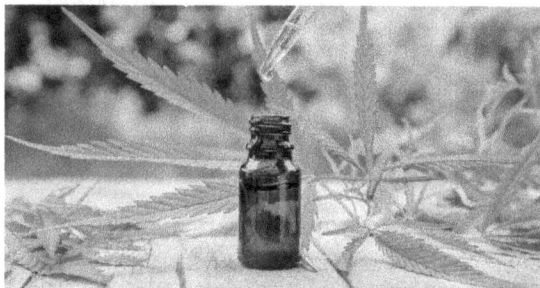

Sublingual

There is also a second way to orally ingest your cannabis. The term sublingual comes from Latin, meaning "under the tongue," and is usually utilized using hard candies and tinctures.

Tinctures have become more and more popular over the years. Maybe it's because the name and the delivery method presents itself as more "medicinal," as opposed to the appearance of edibles being halfway between medicine and candy. I honestly can't even pretend to know how stigmas get attached to things. I'd like to think that we are evolving into a society that can see the potential medical benefits of going the sublingual route, however, I will not be holding my breath on this.

Tinctures, according to our dusty pharmacopeia, are actually alcohol based and not oil based, as you see in retail shops. These drops are meant to be placed under the tongue for optimal absorption in hopes that skipping the road trip through our digestive system, and the hard right turn towards liver conversion, will lead to more of the product making it into the bloodstream.

Research reports that consuming cannabis this way can result in the effects occurring in as little as 20 minutes, lasting between 6-8 hours, and offering bio-availability of 40%–50% of your initial milligram intake.[91] [92]

———

We now know that just chomping down and swallowing an infused hard candy can take up to two hours to kick in, also resulting in the loss of all the original D9THC due to the liver conversion into 11-Hydroxy THC. I usually recommend that people taking hard candy edibles should let it hang out in their mouth for a while. It can't hurt (dentists will disagree), and you may just get your desired effects quicker and with a bit more potency.

But what about those that have genetic differences when it comes to how their body processes drugs?

———

We have all heard the stories about someone that can eat hundreds of mgs of THC and not feel a thing. I had a co-worker that was one of these people. Hudson had pretty much given up on any other method of intake outside of smoking it, and he saw any additional attempts to gain relief from edibles as a waste of money. So, at a company Sunday barbeque I approached him with the idea of trying an edible—but going the sublingual route this time. There was a novel, 25 mg tic tac-like product that was perfect for this kind of experiment. I gave him the low-down on my theory that his liver enzyme was out of whack, and that it changes the way his body processes ingested THC. Hudson shrugged his shoulders and said, "I'm game."

Since it was my idea, I dug the tiny piece of candy out of my stash box and instructed him to let it melt in his mouth for as long as he could stand it. These were the days when processors weren't focused on taste, as they were still struggling with getting their cannabinoid numbers consistent. Therefore, most of the products tasted like bong water.

---

[91] *Human Cannabinoid Pharmacokinetics - PMC (nih.gov)*
[92] *A Systematic Review on the Pharmacokinetics of Cannabidiol in Humans - PMC (nih.gov)*

As a dog day of summer crept along, I had almost forgotten about our morning guinea pig session until I heard the telltale giggle that is unique to an infused edible. Peaking my head out of the kitchen, I saw Hudson shaking what his mama gave him and whistling along with the tune coming out of the speakers as he flipped burgers. "You're feeling it, aren't you," I said with a curious grin.

"This is fantastic Ang. I've never felt weed like this before," he said with elation. Pleased with myself for a successful trial, I had him repeat the reason behind his newfound method of intake to ensure he had it right so he could pass the knowledge on to our patients.

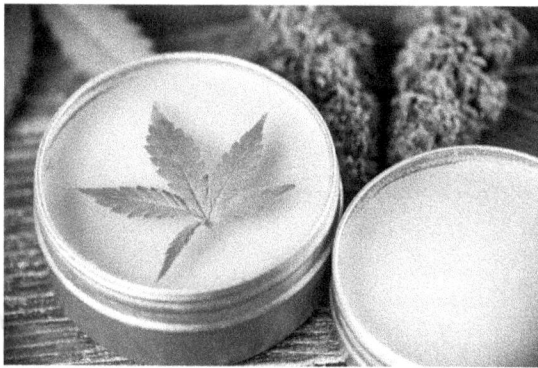

Topicals vs. Patches

By mass, our skin is the human body's largest organ. Ointments, salves, and plant matter have been applied to the human skin since the beginning of time, but the transdermal application of cannabis didn't get any traction until technology caught up during the last third of the 20th century.[93]

Both topical and transdermal patches are applied to the skin, so what is the difference? Topicals target exactly what their name suggests. They are meant for the treatments of medical issues that are on the top of our skin, like rashes. On the other hand, transdermal patches are made to get the intended medicine into the bloodstream. This is a sure way to bypass the digestive tract and any liver conversions during a first pass metabolism, and therefore (in theory) will have greater bioavailability than taking cannabis orally.[94]

Topicals can be lotions, creams, oils, or anything that you rub into your skin. Generally, the effect can be felt in as little as a couple of minutes and can last as long as a couple of hours. The bioavailability isn't great at 5%–10% due to our

---

[93]https://www.ncbi.nlm.nih.gov/pmc/articles/PMC4403087/
[94]https://pubmed.ncbi.nlm.nih.gov/26517407/

mighty skin barrier, but topicals can be great for on-the-go inflammation and surface nerve and joint pain, as it is applied at the source.[95]

Of course, this is assuming the product does not reek like weed. The cannabis industry is still struggling with getting the pot smell out of topicals. We've come a long way, but still have farther to go when it comes to attending to our skin with cannabis. The last thing you want is to do is stink up the joint (pun intended) when you didn't even smoke anything!

I personally am a big supporter of topicals for their skincare benefits alone. Being from a state that is shaped like a mitten, you can imagine how unreasonable the winters are here. Over the years, with a ton of trial and error, I have found that CBD/CBC in a cream-based product does an amazing job at protecting my aging Polish skin.

Research is showing that not only are topicals great for pain caused by inflammation, but they can do some of the heavy lifting when it comes to more serious skin conditions such as wound healing, psoriasis, and melanoma. Granted, these topicals are usually super concentrated variations of FECO (RSO), but still show promise of being a nonintoxicating aid nonetheless.[96]

Transdermal Patches
Even though these patches are not really cost efficient for everyday use, I'm still a groupie of the transdermal patches that are available. They are discreet, low dose, and can help with a wide range of issues. I have often recommended the CBD patches for those that have anxiety about flying, or for those that need a longer relief period than flower or edibles; THC, 1:1's, and other combos are available as well. They are basically nicotine patches, but for cannabis. These little beauties can give anywhere from eight to ten hours of consistent, low dose medicine, and are to be placed on places where your skin is the thinnest.

———

Placement should be on the top of the foot, inside of the wrist, or even on the underside of your arm. This last one is less than desirable due to the fact that the adhesive can be super strong, so it can hurt when you peel it off. The strength of

---

[95]https://www.ncbi.nlm.nih.gov/pmc/articles/PMC6
[96]https://www.potforthepeople.co/skin-conditions

the adhesive is also something to consider when looking to use it on bruised, or paper-thin skin. Another attribute that I like about this method of intake is the fact that if the effects are too strong, or not what you were looking for, you can simply remove the patch and you should be back to good in under an hour. You can also cut the patches in half or quarters in order to dial in the dosage next time around.[97]

I personally use them when I get a tattoo. The last one I got was quite large on my left arm and it took over seven hours to complete it in one sitting. There is no way I could have sat for that long, under that kind of pain, without my trusty patch on the inside of my left wrist.

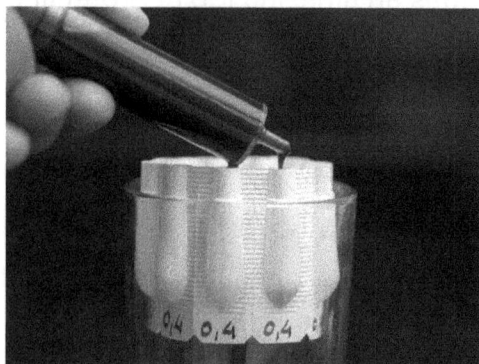

Rectally
That's right folks, cannabis can also be used for and through the back door. I have seen them used for everything from hemorrhoids to rectal cancer, and they even make them for a female's front door.

If you have ever used any type of suppository, you know how messy they can be, and those made from cannabis are no different. They are generally just a mix of coconut oil and FECO (RSO), which is then poured into bullet-shaped molds (you can find these online) to set up in the freezer. Here in Michigan, the dispensaries could not carry them at the time, as all of our products were required to be shelf stable (meaning it couldn't require refrigeration). That being said, I have walked more than a few people through the process of how to make cannabis suppositories for themselves at home after their doctors gave them the go-ahead to try this method of intake.

The feedback from those that have used suppositories is that there is very little buzz, if any at all. Most people say it feels like your body is in a warm bath, and the most unwanted side effect is simply that they are a mess to work with. In theory this is an ideal route for getting high concentrations of cannabis into the

[97]https://www.ncbi.nlm.nih.gov/pmc/articles/PMC6222489/

bloodstream without being metabolized by the liver, and therefore there isn't a conversion from THC to 11-Hydroxy-THC .

Butt (see what I did there), the jury is out on the bioavailability of cannabinoids making it past the membranes in the caboose. According to some of the most recent research, THC itself will not get the job done as one might think. There is a man-made compound of THC called THC-HS (tetrahydrocannabinol-hemisuccinate)[98] that is showing promise as far as absorption rates.

———

So, do suppositories work? Many swear that they do, and it is the only way they could tolerate the high concentrations of cannabis. A person will have a far easier time taking these high doses of cannabis through the basement as opposed to the attic.

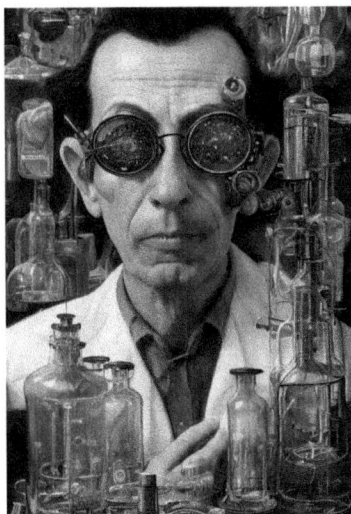

Science!
As we evolve as an industry, more and more smart people will come up with wild inventions, changing our relationship with cannabis forever.

There is the inhaler (just like for asthma) that promises to deliver the right combination of cannabinoids and terps directly to the source without having to smoke anything. As we discussed before, there are certain terpenes that act as a bronchodilator, meaning it helps open up the lungs. It also offers controlled dosing, so you know exactly how much you are intaking with each breath.[99]

———

There is the wide world of nanotechnology, which is exactly like it sounds and then some. Dr. Daniel Stein with Neurology of Cannabis in 2020 wrote: "Scientists are unlocking the potential of treating disease by utilizing nanotechnology and the cannabis plant—diseases like cancer, multiple sclerosis, Parkinson's, diabetes, and serious inflammation. Cannabinoids can be stored inside a nanoparticle and delivered to its intended target without degrading before its controlled

[98] https://www.karger.com/Article/Pdf/489037
[99] https://thisismodernaging.com/cannabis-inhalers/

release. Nanotechnology can help locate and isolate a disease as early as the first few damaged cells; then deliver a targeted cannabinoid to amend the cellular behavior before the damage continues."[100]

And then there is the "smart patch." According to their patent, "The present invention is [a] method of using a smart patch, with analyte testing capabilities, to test a wearer's sweat for the levels of various cannabinoids and delivering at least one other cannabinoid to the user from a reservoir in the patch, to maximize the therapeutic effects according to the user's preferences. A user has a treatment plan with an effective dose. The patch tests the sweat of the user and when it goes outside of the therapeutic range, releases the correct amount of the cannabinoid in the reservoir to return to the therapeutic range, or into a different range specified by the user surrounding the consumption event of a cannabis product through a connected vaporizer."[101]

I will say that the only product to hit the market (so far) that I disapprove of are the infused alcoholic drinks. My skepticism is based upon how quickly booze kicks in versus how slowly it can take to feel the effects of ingested cannabis.

Let's say it's been an ass kicker of a week and you hit your local watering hole on a Friday for a few beers. Your go-to beer is something light on the alcohol content, but you opted for the infused version that carries 10 mgs of THC per bottle. Three beers in and you are just beginning to feel the effects of the first 10 mgs consumed (depending on how quickly the beers go down). You order takeout food, and while waiting you have a fourth beer, bringing your total of consumed mgs to 40—but you're still only feeling the first 10 mgs. Assuming the cottonmouth doesn't have you ordering more beers (or more carryout) than you normally would, you still have 30 mgs waiting for you in the wings. Yes, yes, of course the consumption of anything that gives you a buzz comes with personal responsibility, but with both of these intoxicants working on different timetables, it just feels like you're asking for trouble.

---

[100]https://www.neurologyofcannabis.com/blog/cannabis-nanotechnology/
[101]https://patents.google.com/patent/WO2020084456A1/en

As you continue to read you will see that I am a huge advocate of whole plant medicines and products. Imagine that you have a scoop of cannabinoids, a dollop of terpenes and a dash of flavonoids in that joint in your hand or that tincture under your tongue. When all of these botanical wonders are working together you have what is called the "entourage effect," and this is becoming more of a truth than a theory.

I have always had more questions than a four-year-old at bedtime when it comes to how cannabis works in the body. I have approached many a scientist in hopes of furthering my knowledge of the subject. But unfortunately, there are too many that carry the same up-on-a-pedestal opinion that "if you can't understand it the way I say it the first time, well, then I guess you don't deserve to have this knowledge." I've even had a few tell me that I had no right to do any research on my own, that it is best left to those with a higher education. Both of these examples still rub me the wrong way when I think about them.

So, thank goodness that there are still those that offer explanations at the layman level. I have found that these individuals are secure enough to put aside their ego to truly help us non-STEM people understand the situation. Chuck Kreiman is one of these scientists. He had spent almost two decades in drug discovery/delivery as a medicinal chemist for some huge pharma research groups focusing on neuroscience and cardio-metabolic disorders, prior to focusing on botanical medications. Once on the green side of the pharma fence, he designed and then put into practice a pretty cool delivery system for cannabinoid-based medicines, and now is the director of Indo Laboratories in Massachusetts. In short, this guy knows what he is talking about when it comes to how this plant and its compounds work, and how the human body can get the most bang for its buck. There is an ongoing argument over the idea of whole-plant synergy and whether terpenes/flavonoids really do anything with cannabinoids. In a recent post Chuck summed it up in the best way I have heard yet.

"The way I see it, cannabinoids are still the medicinal star of the show, but they are 'sticky' and poorly behaved from an ADME (ADME stands for 'absorption, distribution, metabolism, and excretion', and describes the disposition of a pharmaceutical compound within an organism)[102] standpoint. While individual

---

[102]https://en.wikipedia.org/wiki/ADME

---

terpenes likely contribute a 'flavor' to the medicinal effects, their purpose is to act as a natural formulation or 'lubricant' to allow the cannabinoids to get to their destination. Actually, terpenes acting as a cardboard boat is a better analogy. That boat can only hold a certain number of packages (THC/CBD) before it starts to dissolve. Once the boat or lubrication is gone, the cannabinoids go back to sticking to everything they come in contact with."

THE ENTOURAGE EFFECT

The entourage effect is the theory that cannabinoids, terpenes, and flavonoids all work better as a whole than working independently. I like to use vitamin C as an example when explaining this to others.

Let's say you are trying to get some vitamin C into your life, and you have the choice between an orange (whole plant) and a vitamin supplement (isolate). The orange is a natural source of protein, fiber, folate, calcium, potassium, in addition to over 90% of your daily requirement for vitamin C. Compare that to the supplement, which only has synthetic fillers for vitamin C to play with. Which would you choose?[103]

Full spectrum vs. Broad spectrum

You will see one of these two terms on just about every CBD product out there. But what is the difference and why does it matter?

Full spectrum means that the product has retained the full range of what was available in the beginning plant matter. These products can carry up to 0.3% of THC, along with the other cannabinoids, and has the potential to pop positive on a drug test.

Broad spectrum, also called "wide" spectrum, is when the product only has some of the plant's original properties. These products will have fewer original terpenes and cannabinoids than full spectrum. Even though these companies try really hard to ensure that zero THC is involved, it can still happen. If you are looking for something that has absolutely no chance of containing THC, isolate is the way to go, as it is straight-up pure CBD. These products are ideal for those that are sensitive to THC and/or those that are concerned about being drug tested.[104]

Isolates vs. Whole Plant

There isn't any difference between CBD or THC that comes from hemp or marijuana. A compound is a compound. But it is the other influencing factors that can change how your body interacts with the compound.

---

[103]https://www.healthline.com/nutrition/oranges#nutrition
[104]https://www.medicalnewstoday.com/articles/full-spectrum-cbd-vs-broad-spectrum-cbd#differences

THE ENTOURAGE EFFECT

The entourage effect is a proposed mechanism by which canabis compounds act synergistically to modulate the overall pstchoactive effects of the plant, primarily by the action of CBD and THC.

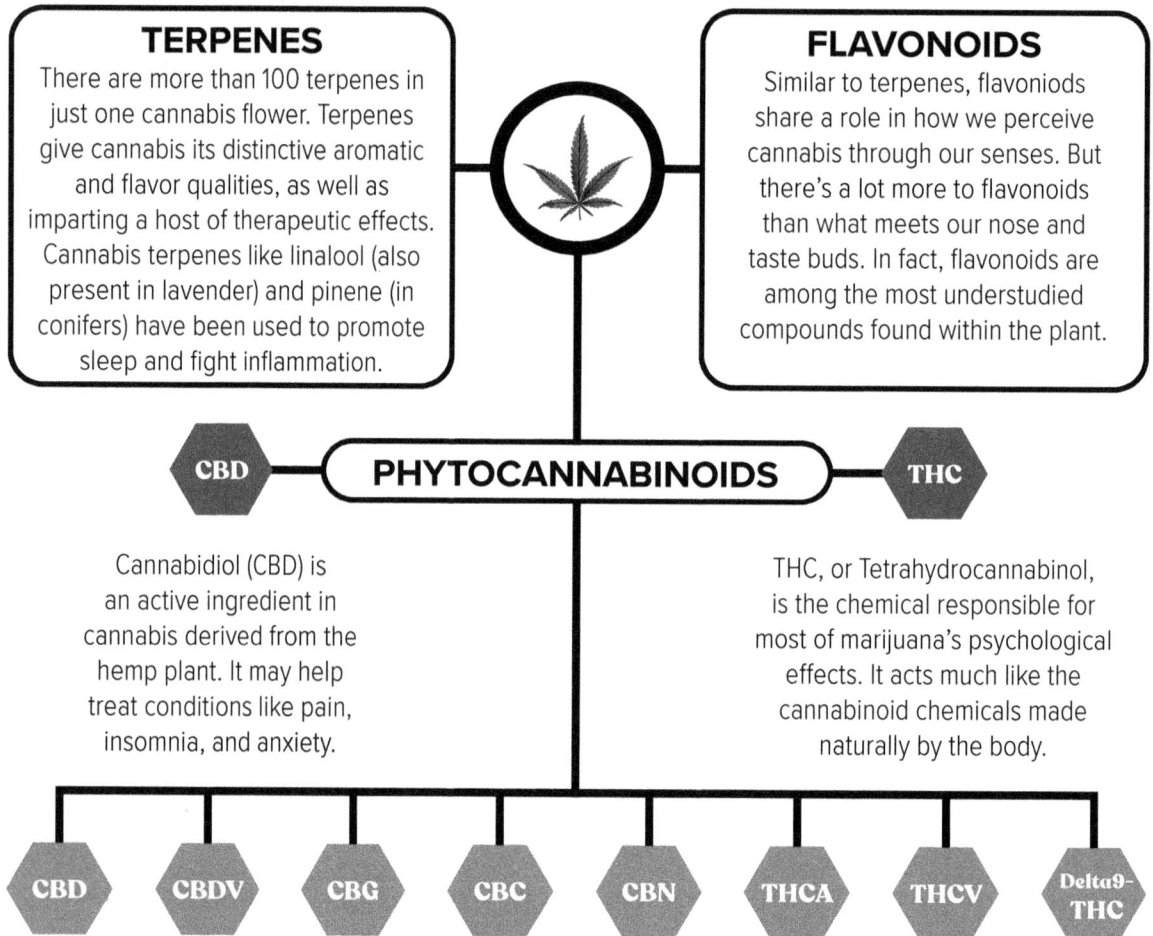

TERPENES

There are more than 100 terpenes in just one cannabis flower. Terpenes give cannabis its distinctive aromatic and flavor qualities, as well as imparting a host of therapeutic effects. Cannabis terpenes like linalool (also present in lavender) and pinene (in conifers) have been used to promote sleep and fight inflammation.

FLAVONOIDS

Similar to terpenes, flavoniods share a role in how we perceive cannabis through our senses. But there's a lot more to flavonoids than what meets our nose and taste buds. In fact, flavonoids are among the most understudied compounds found within the plant.

CBD — PHYTOCANNABINOIDS — THC

Cannabidiol (CBD) is an active ingredient in cannabis derived from the hemp plant. It may help treat conditions like pain, insomnia, and anxiety.

THC, or Tetrahydrocannabinol, is the chemical responsible for most of marijuana's psychological effects. It acts much like the cannabinoid chemicals made naturally by the body.

CBD | CBDV | CBG | CBC | CBN | THCA | THCV | Delta9-THC

Phytocannadinoids or exogenous cannabinoids are plant-derived cannabinoids produced by glandular trichomes covering the surface of the cannabis plant. Trichomes are responsible for producing all of the plant's desirable compounds. More than 100 cannabinoids have been discovered in the cannabis plant. Phytocannabinoids interact with our body's receptors to produce nurerous psychotropic and therapeudic effects. Both plants and animals produce their own cannabinoids, those produced inside the mammalian body are called endocannabinoids. Phytocannabinoids demonstrated above are Cannabidiolic acid (CBDA), Cannbigerol (CBG), Cannabichromene (CBC), Cannabinol (CBN), Tetrahydrocannabinolic acid (THCA), Tetrahydrocannabivarin (THCV), Delta-9-tetrahydrocannabinol (Δ^9-THC)

There are several studies that back up the idea that when the cannabis plant is administered with all of its original properties intact, it not only works better, but it takes lower doses to achieve the same results as a higher-dose isolate.[105]

Of course, science needs to splice and dice individual cannabinoids and terpenes to see what they can and cannot do. But I will tell you that the minute the cannabis plant is pulled apart like this, the magic is lost. You can try to "reintroduce" terpenes and add cannabinoid isolates to the product, but it is never truly the same.

———

I was once sharing a meal with a cannabis processor who was very adamant that his distillate was so strong, nothing else around could compete. I of course disagreed.

I tried to have an educated discussion with him about the differences between his stripped-down THC concentrate and whole plant offerings. He wouldn't hear it. He was convinced that his 90-plus percent THC was the end-all-be-all. So, in true competitive fashion, I challenged him to try hash rosin, as it's the second strongest whole plant product on the market that you can inhale. I would've gone for the big dog FECO but that is more of an ingestion product than inhalation. I didn't want to give him any room to dispute the outcome. Technically you can smoke FECO but my God is it harsh, and a waste of good medicine, in my opinion.

That very night he sent me a text asking what was in the product I asked him to try. "It most certainly must be laced. I have never felt anything like it," he almost whined.

I smugly responded with, "No, no. Nothing like that. What you're feeling is what happens when you keep as much of the plant together as possible. Now would you agree that even though the THC numbers have an almost 30% difference, that the hash rosin is stronger than your sweetheart distillate?" I cannot say I was surprised when, in true spoiled brat fashion, he would not concede or even acknowledge that he may have learned something new from little ol' me.

---

[105]https://www.scirp.org/pdf/PP_2015021016351567.pdf

TESTING

The testing requirements for cannabis are all over the board. While some states have a laundry list of testing requirements, others waive the basic requirement to even just test products for mold. And there are some labs that report only the facts, while others will make the numbers whatever the client wants. This reminds me of my realtor days when having an appraiser in one's pocket could make the sale a bit more favorable for the client.

——

If you find retailers sporting flowers that "tested" out at over 35% THC, there is a really good chance that these are either the overinflated numbers of a shady testing lab, or the grower sprayed their crop with a concentrate to boost its numbers. Unfortunately, both of these deplorable actions are running rampant in our industry.

But honestly, if people didn't put so much stock in high THC potency numbers (which is nonsense), growers would not be spray tanning their incompetence all over their harvest.

Why Test for Terpenes?

I am a staunch advocate for mandatory terpene testing. If you were paying attention to the preceding pages, you now know that terpenes can have all kinds of different effects on a human. By looking at a terpene test you can tell if the product will be sedative, energetic, or even carry potential allergens. Having this knowledge can reinforce your buying confidence when choosing the right cannabis variant for you.

Remediation

As long as we are on the subject of questionable practices, let's talk about remediation. This technique is used to "clean up" any molds or pesticides that a grower may end up with post-harvest. I still remember the first time I saw this come across my desk. An order had come in and it was still missing the bulk flower that we had ordered several weeks ago from a too-big-for-their-britches grower. I pulled up the order in our system and saw under "testing" that their samples had failed five attempts to produce "acceptable limits" of ick. These guys just kept blasting their harvest with radiation and then resubmitting samples in hopes that the 6th time would be a charm.

The problem was described in reporting done by MLive as such: "For instance, a marijuana flower sample could fail safety testing for the presence of banned pathogens, such as E. coli, aspergillus, or salmonella; or for greater than allowed levels of heavy metals, pesticides, yeast and mold, foreign matter or water activity. The producer could then remediate and retest the product as many times as necessary. If and when it passes, labeling isn't required to contain information about the failed tests or notify the customer that product was remediated."[106]

Thankfully, there are people out there that are fighting to make any remediation public knowledge, because right now it isn't. You have no way of knowing if that joint you smoked on Friday night had been zapped over and over again in an attempt to make it safe for human consumption.

Product consistency, on the other hand, is doing much better than it was in the past. There once was a brand that made gingerbread man-shaped gummies that were notorious for both their potency and lack of homogeneity. They contained 100 mg of THC and you never really knew what you were getting unless you ate the entire thing in one sitting. People reported when just eating an arm or a leg of the little guy they could either get nothing or found that they had consumed all 100 mgs.

This is definitely the wrong way to go when you are using cannabis as medicine. Much like how your favorite brand of blue jeans don't need to be tried on with every new pair because you know exactly how they will fit, we should have the same expectations with our cannabis products.

Product consistency and lab testing wasn't always a thing. But at one particular shop that actually did care about the wellbeing of its patients, there was a policy that the initial batch had to be tested before it was decided if the product would make the cut or not. Once they passed the first test, however, the processors pretty much just ran with the same procedure assuming it would all come out the same. This was most definitely not always the case.

---

[106]https://www.mlive.com/public-interest/2022/03/marijuana-regulators-consider-notifying-consumers-if-their-product-failed-testing.html

Cannabis Carl was a well-known vendor for a very popular edible brand back in the day. Their hippy bars were notorious for being consistent, affordable, and having edibles that didn't even taste like weed. A few days after their delivery, Cannabis Carl came bursting through the front door visibly freaked out and headed straight for the offices on the second floor. First reactions were that he overcharged the big guy or screwed up the order somehow. Although not too far off, the ripple effect was an education in itself.

One of the budtenders religiously ate a 150 mg hippy bar every morning before her shift. It was her medicine, so who was I to judge? But on this day, Tina was an absolute mess. As she made her way to the break room to ride out the buzz, everybody racked their brains to try and understand what could've happened. Knowing her tolerance was way up there, it was assumed something else had gone into the mix. Seeing the popular vendor descend the steps from the offices above at that exact moment made collective light bulbs go off above everyone's heads. "What did you do Carl? What did you do to Tina?" the manager asked accusingly. Sweaty in his panic he said, "Get them off the shelf! All of them! Give me every last hippy bar that you have right now!"

It turned out the complacent kitchen staff had accidentally doubled the THC concentration to 300 mgs per bar in that particular batch. Unfortunately for Carl, he found this out the hard way when delivering the famous treats to a shop in Detroit and found that the exact same reaction had happened to some very, very large and very angry business owners. The difference between the two locations was that these guys actually threatened Carl's well-being because of the mistake, leaving him lucky to get out of there unscathed. Phoning it in can be a very real danger to both personal safety and your health in this business folks.

PEOPLE

"Educating the mind without educating
the heart is no education at all."

– Aristotle

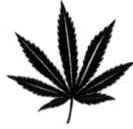

PEOPLE

OUR ENDOCANNABINOID SYSTEM & CANNABIS

You have probably asked yourself at some point how cannabis can possibly work for such a broad range of medical conditions. In the age of very targeted treatments within our healthcare system, anything that claims to help more than a couple of symptoms at once is questioned. I myself even called bullshit on the vast medicinal implications of this plant. This is before I really got into the biological research surrounding cannabis, of course.

Even though cannabis has been around for a very long time, our knowledge about how and why it works in the human body didn't really get a close, hard look until the structure of the most popular phytocannabinoid, THC, was isolated by Mechoulam and Gaoni in 1964. This discovery spurred developments in the research of the Endocannabinoid System (ECS).[107]

Every single one of us has an Endocannabinoid System (ECS)—even our pets have one. Our bodies naturally produce endocannabinoids to interact with certain receptors, and it has been discovered that the cannabis plant, which produces phyto cannabinoids, has a structural similarity to these natural molecules that can stimulate the exact same receptors. This has led to a popular theory that an endocannabinoid deficiency could be the culprit of many medical conditions.

Think of your ECS as a regulator, a mother duck whose job is to keep all her ducklings on track. One of the reasons the cannabis plant can potentially aid in

[107]Crocq MA. History of cannabis and the endocannabinoid system . Dialogues Clin Neurosci. 2020 Sep;22(3):223-228. doi: 10.31887/DCNS.2020.22.3/mcrocq. PMID: 33162765; PMCID: PMC7605027

ENDOCANNABINOID SYSTEM

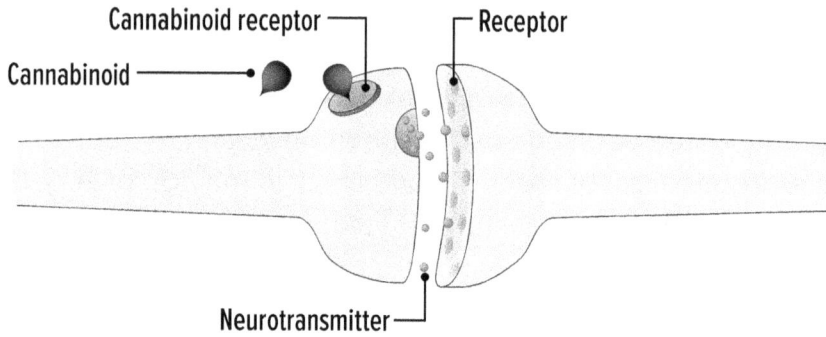

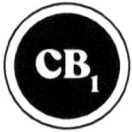

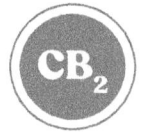

Cannabinoid receptor

Receptor

Cannabinoid

Neurotransmitter

CB₁

CB₂

- Peripheral nervous system
- Central nervous system
- Brain and spinal cord
- Digestive tract
- Pituitary gland
- Thyroid gland
- Adrenal gland
- Muscle cells
- Liver cells
- Fat cells
- Placenta
- Ovaries
- Kidneys
- Ovaries
- Retina
- Lungs
- Sperm

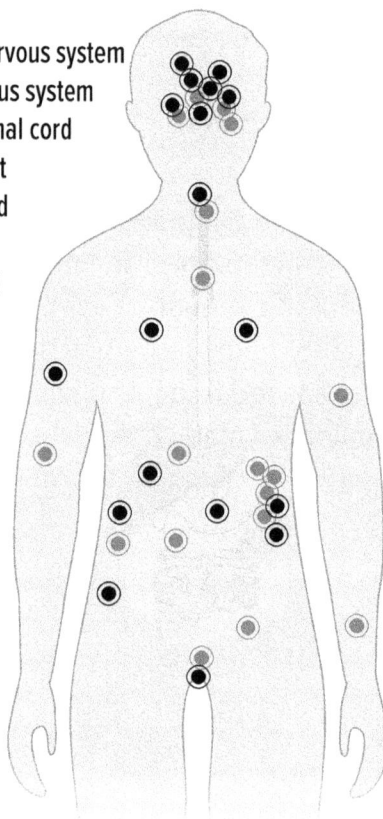

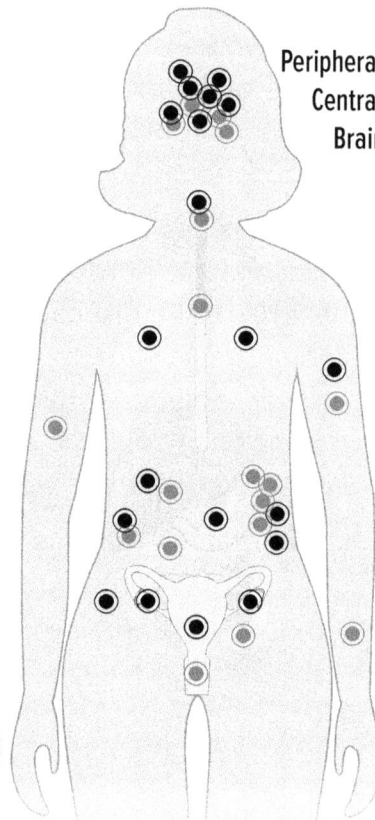

Peripheral nervous system
Central nervous system
Brain and spinal cord
Digestive tract
Pituitary gland
Thyroid gland
Adrenal gland
Muscle cells
Liver cells
Fat cells
Placenta
Ovaries
Kidneys
Ovaries
Retina
Lungs
Sperm

such a wide range of conditions is because it interacts with all of our internal systems. If your nervous system is firing way too hot, your ECS may tell it to calm it down. If your immune system is sluggish and unproductive, your ECS may tell it to get up off its tush and do its job. Our ECS keeps track of these ducklings as they wander off or fall behind and brings them back into the fully functioning fold.

———

The two most popular cannabinoid receptors in current research are the CB1 and CB2. Some of the CB1 receptors are located in the brain, spinal cord, lungs, and kidneys, just to name a few. The CB2 receptors can be found in the immune system, spleen, liver cells, and the nervous system. As research evolves every day, we are finding more and more interactions with these receptors.

According to Dr. Peter Grinspoon from Harvard Medical School, "The 'cannabinoid' receptors in the brain—the CB1 receptors—outnumber many of the other receptor types on the brain. They act like a traffic cop to control the levels and activity of most of the other neurotransmitters.

A second type of cannabinoid receptor, the CB2 receptor, exists mostly in our immune tissues and is critical to helping control our immune functioning, and it plays a role in modulating intestinal inflammation, contraction, and pain in inflammatory bowel conditions. CB2 receptors are particularly exciting targets of drug development because they don't cause the high associated with cannabis that stimulating the CB1 receptors does (which is often an unwanted side effect)."[108]

———

In review, any cannabinoid that pokes the CB1 receptor will have some intoxicating effects. However, if the CB2 receptor is provoked, you will not get that intoxication reaction. And stimulating both of the receptors at the same time can lead to yet another experience. So, knowing which cannabinoids and/or cannabinoid terpene combos interact with which receptors, and how they interact, may just give us some of the answers we have been looking for when it comes to using botanical medicine.

---

[108] https://www.health.harvard.edu/blog/the-endocannabinoid-system-essential-and-mysterious-202108112569

THE MOST COMMON POSITIVE SIDE EFFECTS

After years of feedback from the legions of patients that have crossed my path, three of the most popular positive side effects from cannabis are solid sleep, general relaxation, and movement in their pipes. The first two may not surprise you, as cannabis is well-known for these qualities. But the last one was something I hadn't considered until people began to really speak openly about their cannabis use.

We all know that one of the most common side effects of taking pharmaceuticals is constipation. But some people found that as they used cannabis to either wean off or supplement their medications, they began to consistently take the Browns to the Superbowl again.

THE MOST COMMON NEGATIVE SIDE EFFECTS OF CANNABIS

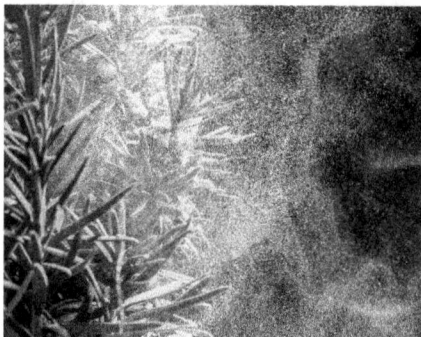

Allergic Reactions

As we all know, introducing nature into our lives can be both a blessing and a curse—just ask anyone with seasonal allergies. A person can absolutely have an allergic reaction to cannabis.

Cannabis does not have to interact with other substances, such as prescribed drugs, to be harmful. Whether suffering a reaction from constantly overindulging in THC, or reacting to certain terpenes, allergic side effects from consuming cannabis are a possibility. "Linalool is a major constituent of cannabis and can be a very weak allergen if an allergic reaction occurs at all. However, linalool autoxidizes on air exposure, and the oxidation products can cause contact allergy. If a person who develops an allergy to these byproducts inhales linalool via concentrates, a strong anaphylaxis, or systemic allergic reaction which includes the familiar symptoms of hyperventilation, hives, and itchiness, can likewise occur."[109]

So even though most of us will feel a calming sensation from encountering lavender in nature, inhaling it in concentrated form at high temperatures can be totally different, and sometimes will have harmful outcomes.

---

[109]https://terpenesandtesting.com/category/science/cannabis-allergies/

A person really has to be aware of their own bodies and heed the warnings. If you know that you are allergic or sensitive to dairy, you scan labels to ensure that you won't be doing yourself in. The same line of thinking has to go into any natural airborne allergies you might have, as the very same terpenes that are found in these plants can also be found in the cannabis you are consuming, especially when smoking or vaporizing your flower or concentrates. This is yet another reason why terpene testing should be mandatory at the state level, especially in the medical markets.

Cannabinoid Hyperemesis Syndrome (CHS)

CHS is fairly new and is confusing both the medical community and the consumer. While the scientific world isn't quite sure of the cause, the cannabis industry has theories that it is caused by crappy growing processes, including monsterous pesticides and fertilizers being sprayed directly on the plant as well as added to the soil.

How can this be allowed for human consumption? Are we not supposed to pass all cannabis products through a staunch testing procedure? Unfortunately, this procedure isn't worth very much when some unethical testing labs have their palms greased by slimy growers.

> "Cannabinoid Hyperemesis Syndrome is characterized by chronic cannabis use, cyclic episodes of nausea and vomiting, and frequent hot bathing. Cannabinoid Hyperemesis Syndrome occurs by an unknown mechanism."[110]

These side effects are different from those reported from over doing it with edibles. In fact, many of the effects of CHS can be absent for years (especially if a person abused cannabis as an adolescent), and then rear its ugly head once a person begins to indulge in cannabis again. According to the study quoted above, not only THC, but CBD and CBG, may also play a role in CHS.

---

[110]*Galli JA, Sawaya RA, Friedenberg FK. Cannabinoid hyperemesis syndrome. Curr Drug Abuse Rev. 2011 Dec;4(4):241-9. doi: 10.2174/1874473711104040241. PMID: 22150623; PMCID: PMC3576702*

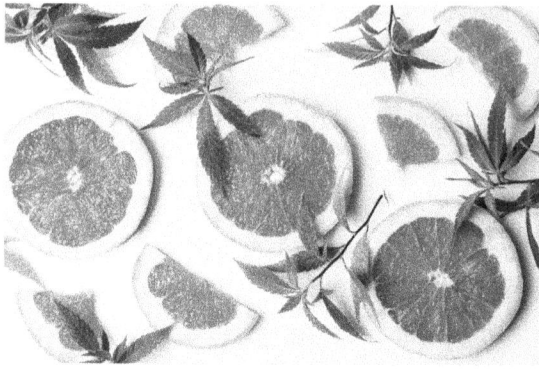

Drug Interactions

While we are still on the subject of the negatives of cannabis, let's discuss the reality of cannabis and drug interactions.

———

Cannabis does have drug interactions. Please understand this statement. We have been so conditioned to leaving this up to our doctors and pharmacists that most of us will not take the time to look into it ourselves. We most definitely do not have this luxury when it comes to cannabis. This interaction can cause a drug to be far less or way more potent than intended, and it is up to personal responsibility to ensure you are doing everything you can to protect yourself.

A very basic way to know if your current (and future) pharmaceuticals will have an interaction with cannabis is to watch for a "grapefruit warning" on your pill bottles. This sour citrus dances with the same metabolizing liver enzyme that we had spoken about earlier in regard to edibles. "Grapefruit juice decreases the activity of the cytochrome P450 3A4 (CYP3A4) enzymes that are responsible for breaking down many drugs and toxins."[111] Some may think that you would have to drink gallons of the stuff in order for it to have an effect. Think again.

> "One whole fruit or 200 milliliters of grapefruit juice (a bit less than one cup) can block the CYP3A4 enzymes and lead to toxic blood levels of the drug."[112]

Blood thinners and medications for epilepsy are famous for having this warning attached to their bottles. Let's say that you have been taking the same drug for years to keep your seizures at bay, and it's working, but you would like to try to introduce cannabis into your healthcare regimen. The very last thing you want is to start having seizures again because you didn't do your due diligence.

It would also be wise to ask your doctor if any newly proposed medications carry this warning prior to them prescribing it. The conversation could go some-

---

[111]https://www.drugs.com/article/grapefruit-drug-interactions.html
[112]https://www.drugs.com/article/grapefruit-drug-interactions.html

thing like this: "I would like to start you on ABC medication for your migraines," your doctor says. You can respond with, "Does ABC come with a grapefruit warning? I use CBD and I know it carries the same warnings as a grapefruit interaction." If your new medication has just phoned into the pharmacy, be sure to ask the same question so everyone is on the same page.

There is an available search engine to check if a certain medication interacts with cannabis. I have not been given permission to add the actual link, so I will tell you to search Penn State's website (wink).

———

Doing Your Own Digging

Let's be honest. Anyone can find research to fit their own narrative. If you are against cannabis, there are plenty of studies that show the harm in, let's say, inhaling cannabis. Inhaling combustion with all of its carcinogens isn't good for anyone. We all know this. But on the other hand, there are studies showing that it can actually open up your lungs when the right combo of cannabinoids/terpenes are involved, and therefore is potentially beneficial for those with lung issues. I know, I know. It sounds crazy, but this information is leading processors to inventions such as an inhaler that delivers a specific cannabinoid/terpene profile directly to the source.[113]

Unfortunately, these inconsistencies are everywhere when it comes to the research of cannabis. I blame the bulk of funding favoring the negative attributes of cannabis, not to mention the research monopoly the United States has been under for over 80 years. But we Americans can also sometimes forget that we are not the only educated nation in the world. Several countries have been studying this plant, its compounds, and its effects for decades on end.

———

I was once hired to do some cannabis education for a local processor whose head honcho was an environmental scientist. I liked the person. I respected the person's opinions, but I can only imagine the look on my face when this person tried to condition me to the idea that Europeans provided nothing but "junk sci-

---

[113]https://pubmed.ncbi.nlm.nih.gov/36737540/

ence." After this very uneducated, ego-driven statement, I unfortunately began to see one of my favorite people in a different light.

So do your own research. Afterall, who knows what you have going on mentally, physically, and emotionally better than you! Form your own opinions about what the science has to say about cannabis and your afflictions. And then print out the studies and go have educated discussions with your doctors. They don't have to like that you are doing your own research (most won't). But they do have to respect your right to play an active part in your own healthcare.

What we know (and don't know) about this plant literally changes and evolves every single day, and as someone who has fallen down at least one cannabis rabbit hole a day for the past 12 years, I can tell you that it can be confusing and overwhelming as hell. But I have found a few rules of thumb to follow to help sort out the knowledge from the nonsense.

> **Rule of Thumb:** Consider the source — If someone came at you with the idea that the earth is flat and was adamant that it simply must be true because they found it on the internet, well, you'd laugh at them (I hope). Ideally you will want double-blind, peer-reviewed human study status, but science doesn't start there, it starts with compounds and animals. Yes, yes. I understand that we are not animals and that research using animal models can be easy to discredit. But outside of the obvious risk of using unknown substances on humans, do you know why science uses animals?

According to Stanford, some animals are so biologically similar to us to the point where we share more than 98% of the same DNA with mice.[114] Animals are also vulnerable to many of the same health conditions and issues as we are. And with a shorter life span than humans, researchers can study them through a few generations to see how these diseases progress and how they interact biologically. Think of it as science taking baby steps when researching cannabis.

So that being said, do not discount findings that don't meet all of the above requirements, as they are very much a part of the process when it comes to drug research. I have found national scientific research sites, major medical universities, and medical journals to be credible when it comes to tearing this plant apart. I mean aren't these the same entities that educate our future doctors and scientists? And if we were fortunate enough to have been taught how to read, why

---

[114]https://med.stanford.edu/animalresearch/why-animal-research.html

---

should we have to acquire tens of thousands of dollars in student debt to learn from the same public materials?

Rule of Thumb: Look at the dates — As I said before, we are just getting into the nitty gritty of the cannabis plant, and even though the research paper may only be a few years old, it could definitely be outdated and/or debunked. The most recent papers and studies are your best bet.

Rule of Thumb: Anecdotal evidence — We know what opinions are like and how everybody has one. I generally shy away from opinion pieces and blogs. While you don't have to convince the hundreds of thousands of us using cannabis that it works as medicine, using solid scientific research references will ensure that even the naysayers cannot just brush it off as just an opinion.

When coming across these offerings, scan the document for links to the actual studies they are talking about and then reference my first rule by making sure it comes from a credible source. If the publication lacks solid references, I wouldn't put too much stock in what it has to say.

MEDICAL PROFESSIONALS

At some point, probably around the time house calls ceased, doctors simply stopped engaging with their patients. Regardless of whether the blame lies with liability insurance, overcrowding, or countless other excuses, the end result is the same. Patients have been degraded to nothing more than a medical file.

By ignoring the human connection with their patients, the bulk of healthcare providers have neglected this key part of what it means to heal. Today's doctors are trained not to get involved, and to not share their personal experiences, even if they can help their patients by doing so. This frustration of not being seen or listened to is one of the main reasons so many have shunned traditional medication and turned to cannabis.

The anti-cannabis people out there love to say that there is not enough research to even humor condoning its use. This could not be further from the truth. If you are one of these people, I challenge you to go to PubMed and simply put "cannabis" in the search bar. As I write this you will find 30,145 results.

As you can imagine, you will get a variety of topics such as different diseases, the endocannabinoid system, and drug abuse. Unfortunately, reefer madness is still alive and well when it comes to where the funding for cannabis research ends up. According to reports on cannabis research grants and funding in the US between 2000 and 2018 "most of the money went to studies focusing on the potential harms of the recreational drug. The U.S. National Institute on Drug Abuse (NIDA), the single biggest source of funds, spent far more money to research cannabis misuse and harmful effects than on the therapeutic benefits of cannabis and cannabis-derived chemicals. And although overall funding for cannabis research in the U.S. has been rising steadily, the money to explore cannabis medical treatments isn't growing as fast as funding for research on harms."[115]

———

I get it. I really do. It only took us 80 plus years to get to where we are now with cannabis. Yes, there are concerns and considerations to be made, as there are with any drug, but as a medical professional you cannot ignore that these compounds were deemed medically useful for hundreds of years prior to the political damning of the plant. You also cannot turn your nose up at the sound research coming from the exact same research and teaching institutions that your medical education is rooted in. Where's your sense of curiosity? What happened to your desire to help others with your knowledge? I personally find that when a doctor brushes off or mocks cannabis research and its potential as medicine, it is not only shortsighted to the point of negligence, but lazy.

I also understand the potential for liability when dealing with pot and your patients. Every health system out there has a wide variety of restraints on its worker bees, even if those gag orders can harm the patient.

I always add cannabis under the "current drugs" on any medical forms. I had an appointment with a new neurologist, and after scanning over my records, she asked if I had a medical marijuana card. I informed her that I did and she visibly relaxed. She told me that she couldn't discuss cannabis or even consider its interaction with my disease unless I had the card. Shocked and irritated all at once, I asked how that line of thinking helps people who just want to ask questions and learn about cannabis for their condition? I got a noncommittal shoulder shrug and a, "it doesn't."

---

[115] https://medium.com/illumination/bias-in-cannabis-research-focuses-on-harmful-effects-f16c7c87e7b1

I have found that doctors will almost always show their true colors when alternative medications are brought up during a visit. They are either an optimistic orange and give-it-a-shot green, or a closed-minded maroon and a narcissistic navy. It is the latter colors that can hinder your medical care—your quality of life. These are the types of medical professionals that are so closed off to anything but their own set-in-stone opinions, that they forget that they work for the patient. Just recently I dismissed a neurologist for telling me that he would only treat my migraines and not my CMT or the nerve damage I picked up from a cage inserted in my spine. As if my health conditions were an à la carte menu he could just pick and choose from.

I have "fired" more than one doctor for this kind of behavior, and to my enjoyment, the look is always astonishment. This may seem harsh to some and bitter to others. But, when these encounters land you on the "difficult patient" list and you get even worse treatment for standing up for yourself, for standing up for the quality of your healthcare, you can't blame a girl for trying to change things in the only way she knows how.

TALKING TO YOUR FAMILY

This can be a daunting task, for sure. Everyone has their own set of beliefs about not only the legal usage of cannabis, but how it will affect both the afflicted and their loved ones. I always encourage people to bring any concerned family members with them or invite them to sit in on a consultation call. I have sat with mothers, sons, neighbors and even a priest or two, in an effort to educate everyone involved. I also recommend that any willing or able family members should try the same dosage of the product as the patient (one priest declined). I find this helps to not only ease their anxiety about cannabis as medicine, but it gives both the patient and the concerned party a better sense of what the afflicted is going through.

Especially in the case of cancer, I try to help the whole family. Let's say that Mom has come down with stage two breast cancer. The world stops for everyone in the family. The focus is 100% on her treatment options, and rightfully so. But we can't forget that Dad hasn't slept a wink since the diagnosis or that her sister has taken on the domestic duties of the home that are beyond her physical capabilities, yet she won't stop trying. By offering a topical for her sister's bad hip or a CBD tincture for Dad to help manage the stress, cannabis can aid this family unit in being the best they can be in caring for Mom.

Talking to Your Kids

I am the last one to tell you when to talk to your kids about cannabis, or any drug for that matter. You know your offspring best. You know their maturity levels, their influences, and their environments. And there isn't anything saying that you can only have "the talk" once. I urge you to readdress the topic as many times as you deem necessary. Cannabis is not going anywhere and the more everyone knows the better.

———

The business of weed has been around these parts since my kid was in middle school, yet we really didn't have "the talk" until she went to high school. Granted, when she was younger there wasn't the ocean of different cannabis products that we have today. With the evolution from homemade pot brownies to 200 mg candy bars with almost identical packaging as common store brands, I knew the responsible thing to do was to give her as much of my cannabis knowledge as she could absorb.

So, one day after school we sat down, and I put her through the "plant" portion of my cannabis retail training. We covered terpenes, cannabinoids, edibles, and the packaging of these products, as well as what FECO was used for and that, in fact, the amber colored syringe was not black tar heroin.

Questions were asked and answered that day, and even though kiddo is an adult now, we still have hearty conversations about new cannabis research, pot politics, and spot-on stoner memes.

Kids in the House

There is a very real, and completely preventable, problem: parents are not doing enough to keep cannabis away from the little ones. Cannabis is a drug. I simply do not understand why parents are not treating it with the same respect as their prescriptions and booze. You put safety locks on your cabinets containing chemicals, you keep your alcohol up high and out of reach like your pills. But you'll leave the pot gummies on the counter?

This is not an adult-access issue. This is not a packaging issue. This is a piss-poor parenting issue. If your child gets into the whiskey, it is your fault. If your child gets into your pills, it is your fault. But if your child gets into your weed, it turns into a pot shop-proximity or packaging problem? Knock it off. Stop trying to shift the responsibility. Do better by your kids.

DRUG TESTING – ON THE JOB AND ON THE ROAD

One of the most common questions retailers get is, "Will I pass a drug test if I'm just taking CBD?" Let us think back to the explanation of spectrums vs. isolates in CBD products. If your CBD gummies or tincture are either broad, wide, or full spectrums, there is always the possibility of trace amounts of THC and therefore the potential to pop hot on a test. But if your chosen product is made with isolates, then I'd say you're pretty safe.

> "According to Quest Diagnostics Director of Science and Technology, Barry Sample, CBD likely won't show up on a drug test: 'If the product contains only CBD and has had the THC removed, then an individual being tested would not be expected to test positive for marijuana or marijuana metabolite.' In other words, marijuana drug tests screen for THC, not CBD."[116]

Now when it comes to mandatory drug tests, many cry foul when a company requires THC drug testing using the argument of local legality. After all, they don't care if you have beers on the weekend, or an open script for heavy painkillers, as long as you can do your job without risk to the company or your fellow employees. Yet when it comes to marijuana, even if you are a medical marijuana card holder, there is often a hard line in the sand against it. And for the most part, for good reason.

Would you want your surgeon stoned before your operation? Do you want that gravel-hauler driver that shares the road with you all grassed up? Would you want your babysitter high watching your terrible-two toddler? I think not.

But there is also a flip side. That surgeon may take a low dose edible before bed to ensure he is properly rested. That truck driver may take a few drops of a CBD tincture that has a splash of THC in it for his bad back. That babysitter may take a microdose as a part of her morning regimen to combat anxiety instead of the tweaker Adderall. None of these examples will render these professionals stoned, and they are using cannabis as medicine—responsibly.

———

There are so many varying degrees of "intoxication" when it comes to cannabis. You may be someone who occasionally takes a gummy to help shut your

---

[116]https://www.usdrugtestcenters.com/drug-test-blog/181/can-you-fail-a-drug-test-due-to-cbd.html

head off at night and by morning you only feel well rested. And then there are those that huff on a vape pen all day, every day. Both of these examples will pop hot on a drug test. Because THC is stored in our fat cells, cannabis will hang around in our system much, much longer than the buzz does.

Ex: You enjoy a few cocktails over Labor Day weekend and the thought of failing a roadside sobriety test on the following Tuesday just isn't realistic. But if you smoke a joint on the same weekend and are subjected to a roadside swab on the way to dropping your kids off at school three weeks later, you will fail the test. So, even though the buzz is long gone, you are now being charged with driving while intoxicated and child endangerment.

The type of test, how often, and how much THC you use, has a lot to do with how long you will be coming in hot on a drug test.

"Research on the amount of time a test can detect cannabis shows a wide range of averages. Research from 2017 estimates a detection window for a single cannabis cigarette of about 3 days."

The same study emphasizes that detection windows vary and depend on how often a person smokes.

It showed:
- For someone smoking cannabis for the first time, tests may detect it for about 3 days.
- In someone who smokes cannabis three or four times per week, the detection window is 5–7 days.
- For people who smoke cannabis once a day or more, tests may detect it in their system for 30 days or longer.

Detection windows also depend on the kind of test a person undertakes. General estimates for various cannabis tests are as follows:
- Urine tests can detect cannabis in the urine for approximately 3–30 days after use.
- Saliva tests can detect cannabis for approximately 24 hours after use. Some saliva tests have detected cannabis for up to 72 hours.
- Hair tests are the most sensitive tests, detecting THC for up to 90 days after use. However, these tests are testing the oil in skin that transfers to hair, and so they may occasionally show a false positive. A person who comes into contact with a THC user could, theoretically, test positive on a hair test.
- Blood tests can only detect THC for 3–4 hours.[117]

[117] https://www.medicalnewstoday.com/articles/324315#failing-a-drug-test

Technology and science must catch up sooner rather than later when it comes to cannabis intoxication. It is imperative that testing for marijuana, roadside or not, be as precise as other impairment tests. People are still having their lives ruined by inaccurate drug testing, and it has to stop. As it stands now, positive test results do not equal intoxication. Read that again.

But if you are someone who likes to brag that you are a better driver when stoned: you are a part of the problem, you deserve the ticket. Nobody should ever, ever drive under the influence of anything that alters your cognition or your reaction time.

CANCER

"Prostate, lung, and colorectal cancers account for an estimated 43% of all cancers diagnosed in men in 2020. For women, the three most common cancers are breast, lung, and colorectal, and they will account for an estimated 50% of all new cancer diagnoses in women in 2020."[118]

Cannabis research regarding cancer has begun to flourish in recent years. There are several studies to support the use of cannabinoids to combat the side effects of chemo, but others that show cannabis can cause more harm, so please do your due diligence and do your own research before starting cannabis.[119]

—

A few years back I was informed upon walking into work that in less than 30 minutes I was to be interviewed to address the topic of the growing relationship between cannabis and cancer.[120]

In the words of Clark Griswold, "If I woke up tomorrow with my head sewn to the carpet, I wouldn't be more surprised than I am right now." Did I know the subject matter well enough to speak about it? Yes. I had this conversation at least five times a week. Was I scared to death about being in front of the camera, and do I loathe surprises of this nature? Yes, and yes.

---

[118] *https://www.cancer.gov/about-cancer/understanding/statistics*
[119] *https://www.potforthepeople.co/cancers*
[120] *https://www.imdb.com/title/tt8456536/*

So aside from cursing myself for wearing a hoodie to work that day, there was nothing else to do but handle the situation as I would any other patient interaction. Once done with giving my two cents, I was to act out a consultation with a cancer patient for the blinding lights in the room. Little did I know that my acting partner that day would become a source of strength for me in the future.

———

Millie had woken one day with a cancerous tumor the size of a bowling ball in her right breast. I am not exaggerating the size, nor how quickly it evolved. Even though she was a retired nurse from one of the largest hospitals in the state, she had far greater faith in alternative medicine than she did in the "pill mills," as she would put it. Millie was using a wide variety of alternative approaches when we met; everything from immunotherapies to mistletoe was thrown at the ticking time bomb in her chest. And like most baby boomers, she had only tried some grass in college and Cousin Eddie's pot brownies during one strange camping trip.

She wanted to learn it all (and take it all), as she was on hourglass time. This sense of urgency (as if the cancer wasn't enough) came from her oncologist, who pretty much told her to get her affairs in order. The doctor's reasoning was that the tumor was so large that they would never get clean margins (get it all out), and then they wouldn't have enough skin to close the space. Finding this unacceptable and absolutely certain that there were still more treatments to try, Millie embraced cannabis.

While Millie was out there looking for a second opinion, she began to use a topical for the skin over the breast, in addition to a tincture so strong that it demands respect. Thankfully, she had a really elevated tolerance for concentrated cannabis and the tincture didn't faze her much. In fact, at one point she was looking for something to help her sleep, even though she was putting away over 2000 mgs of THC daily. How's that for a natural tolerance!

By the grace of God, she had found a doctor in Florida that not only was willing to do the surgery (meaning the attempt wouldn't ruin his reputation), but was confident that he had enough to work with to close afterwards. Millie was both excited and terrified all at once. See, Millie was afraid to fly—she had never done it before. There are no words to do justice to the emotions that must have consumed this woman as she boarded a flight to try and save her own life.

Within a few days after she had the surgery, Millie called me with a voice so elated that I cried at the sound of it. "The surgeon did everything that he said he would! He got the whole tumor out with clean margins and had more than enough skin to close up shop!"

Millie had fought for her life, and she won.

———

After a few weeks in recovery at an Airbnb just outside of Miami, she was cleared to come home and couldn't wait for her next appointment with the same oncologist that gave her a death sentence just months before.

Oh, what I wouldn't give to have been a fly on the wall for the following discussion! Hearing that Millie didn't take her "advice" and took her mortality into her own hands, the doctor became hostile towards her. "Bet you can't put your arms above your head. You do know you'll never be able to put coffee cups away again, don't you?" Millie said the doctor jeered at her.

"So, I gave her one of my famous shit-eating grins, the one I reserve for the extra special jerks and threw both of my arms up over my head. I even gave her a little wave while my fingers reached for the sky," Millie told me in a mischievous tone.

"That's fantastic! Ha-ha. What was her response to that?" I asked, as I love when over-inflated egos lose some air.

"You're going to love this one. She said she would no longer treat me. That she wasn't going to have a patient that wouldn't take her direction, even if it did save their lives."

I'm pretty sure I broke a record somewhere for the most curse words per minute. "She said that to your face?! Please tell me that you went scorched earth on this lady," I begged.

"No. Part of me really, really wanted to—the old me would've burned the building to the ground for sure—but I now know that it wouldn't change anything. So, I just laughed. And laughed and laughed some more until she left the room. The life that I saved, my life, has no energy left for anger. I only have energy for the good from here on out." Millie said.

Whenever my life seems to get overwhelming or viciously unfair, I think of Millie. I think of the amount of sheer courage it takes to fight for your life. Some are squabbles, some are battles, and some are all out war. But to come away from these encounters with a new perspective, an inclination to be a better human ... that is what it means to evolve.

DEMENTIA

The National Institute of Aging defines dementia as a blanket term to cover a variety of mental afflictions and it ... is the loss of cognitive functioning—thinking, remembering, and reasoning—to such an extent that it interferes with a person's daily life and activities. Some people with dementia cannot control their emotions, and their personalities may change."[121]

Up close and personal, dementia is scary and heart wrenching all at the same time. The person that you knew and loved is past the point of no return and there isn't a damn thing anyone can do about it.

Every now and then it feels like nothing short of divine intervention when a consultant is paired up with a patient. It's as if the cannabis-confused stranger in front of you was meant just for you. Sometimes it's because you both share the same medical condition, or life experience, or it could be as insignificant as commiserating over your local sports teams. This story is about how an 80-something-year-old man taught me how to see beyond my initial reactions and left a mark on my heart.

"Hi loser," Stu said with a crooked smile.

Oh boy, I thought, am I really starting my day with degradation? I replied with a level tone, "Now how would you know such a thing when we just met?" Stu leaned in a little closer, as my co-workers within ear shot stopped what they were doing to see if I was going to make this a teachable moment or if I forgot to pack my patience that morning. "Your shirt. I can see you are a fan of our loser baseball

---

[121]*https://www.nia.nih.gov/health/what-is-dementia*

team. That makes you a loser too." I couldn't help but smile at this gentleman's attempt to be charming. Testing our communication boundaries I said, "Well, are you one of those diehards that have been dedicated to our football team since the beginning of time? Because if you are, that makes you an even bigger loser than me." With a shared chuckle, and the staff returning to their tasks disappointed that I didn't snap, we both agreed that our teams were the worst and moved on to the matter at hand.

Stu's bride, as he lovingly referred to her, was stuck in the nightmare that is dementia. Even though she was becoming more and more violent every day, the family decided to release her from the hospital, whose method of treatment was to strap her to a bed and feed her the highest concentrations of sedatives known to man. With tears in his eyes, he was bordering on begging for something, anything to help her. Her pain levels weren't the issue, in fact she didn't take any painkillers at all, but solid sleep was.

The less his wife rested the more likely she was to beat and batter the family in the home.

Gently, I asked Stu if she had a sweet tooth, as this would help me to know if tinctures (which sounded like it would be a nightmare to administer) or sugary edibles would be better. "Sometimes I think that she loves chocolate more than she loves me," Stu said, having regained his composure. Not really trusting that any intake recommendations would make it back to the family unchanged, I wrote down the instructions for him to take home. With a "see ya loser," Stu left the shop with a spring in his shuffle.

———

Not three hours later, Stu had returned with his daughter and son-in-law, who were pretty combative about my recommendations and Stu's purchases. It wouldn't be the first time I had been blamed for "taking advantage" of an elderly patient for pushing them into buying the wrong thing. It's almost always by family members who wanted pop-pop or gam-gam to bring home super high milligram stuff for them.

They explained the family's situation again and were adamant that the milligrams I advised Stu to start with weren't even close to what they wanted for her. "She needs to be drugged. She needs to be sedated at all times," urged Stu's daughter who was bruised from yesterday's battle with her mom.

And there it was. I was automatically protective of both Stu, his bride, and my recommendation. Are these people actually asking me to recommend something that will render this poor woman immobile? Oh hell no. "Cannabis is about quality of life. It is not meant to induce zombie-like reactions. I mean, isn't that the whole reason you discharged her from the hospital?" I clapped back. After a very heavy and long pause, Stu's daughter, Lynne, revealed herself to be a nurse. A nurse that had seen traditional medicine fail her family, and much like her father hours earlier, was just about begging for an alternative solution.

It instantly made perfect sense that the woman in front of me was a caretaker of others. It also made me feel a bit better knowing that her mother was discharged from the hospital and released into her care. Lynne had a very old soul. She was one of those formidable females that demanded respect and attention as soon as she entered the room. There was zero doubt that this woman was the matriarch of her family. I betcha she got it from her mama.

———

And now it was my turn to beg.

I pleaded with them to try the initial purchase, and with Lynne being a nurse and ever mindful of drug interactions, she could adjust different ratios and milligram amounts. I expressed my hope that they would land on the right combination of cannabinoids to calm her mother, but not knock her out.

About a week later, Stu returned with his now endearing greeting of "hi loser" and his freshly scratched and days-old bruise-covered daughter. Lynne reported that they tried a few different combinations without any change in the violent attacks and ended up giving her half of the chocolate bar in one sitting.

I froze.

"You're kidding?" came out of my mouth before I could stop it. It didn't help that I still had it stuck in the back of my mind that these folks just wanted her completely comatose. But before I could scold her for being so reckless, she said with a shrug of her shoulder, "it didn't faze her." Unable to find another statement, I said again "you've got to be kidding me." Both Stu and Lynne confirmed that while she didn't move around the house as much during the intoxication period, her verbal abuse continued and they still couldn't get close, as Lynne's scratches attested to. But they both agreed that it was better than before and wanted to continue using cannabis as treatment.

I immediately became uncomfortable with the conversation, as I knew what the next question was going to be. "Do you have anything stronger?" asked Stu with that hope in his eyes again.

I generally don't recommend RSO to those without cancer or very specific directions from their doctor, but outside of offering that the woman eat several candy bars a day, RSO was the strongest product in the place. I explained why the whole plant concentrate may work better (and differently) than the distillate-infused candy and repeated the dosage and a stern warning to be overly cautious when it came to the amber colored syringe. I also offered the advice of only buying one, because all of this trial and error can get expensive. They both agreed and left with one RSO syringe and another chocolate bar as a "treat" for her.

——

Another couple of weeks had passed before I saw the father and daughter duo in the lobby again. My first thought was that the RSO was just way too much for her and tried to stuff away my "I told you so" speech. But it happened that I returned to my simply shocked "are you kidding me" response when they told me that they made a "sandwich" out of the RSO and candy bar. "Kinda like a smore. She always loved smores," Stu said with a touch of nostalgia in his voice. At this point I am trying to do both the math on how many milligrams she took and find any words at all for the situation.

Now I've seen ridiculous tolerances for cannabis in those that consistently over-partake and in those that take high doses of painkillers for decades, but this lady took the cake.

I was rendered speechless.

They started out by giving her a couple of pieces of chocolate periodically during the day as a reward for good behavior or a bribe for better behavior. They then took what was left of the chocolate and literally squished a quarter gram of RSO between the pieces right before bed. According to Amy, for the first couple of days it was touch and go. Sometimes the candy worked in curbing her violent attacks, and sometimes she wanted nothing to do with her "treats" and would just rage on. True to her calling, Lynne had been keeping a journal of all of her mom's vitals with the different dosages, ratios, and products up to this point.

Stu jumped in on the storytelling by saying that once it became routine, she began lashing out less. Her mean-spirited outbursts were shorter and at times almost mumbled like she really didn't want to say them in the first place. Still floored by the amount of cannabis this woman can take in a sitting, I returned to consultant mode by remembering that there actually was a smores-like chocolate bar and offered to substitute it for the original one. For my efforts I got a warm, "thank you for paying attention" smile from Lynne, and a wink and a "thanks loser" from Stu.

We stayed in contact and sometimes I would even visit Stu at the curb when his wife made the trip with them. Every so often, she would have a morning or an afternoon where she was manageable in public, or mentally present enough to enjoy a Sunday car ride like the old days when their love was new.

I also got a few more minutes to talk smack with Stu about our cursed sports teams. One such visit even included my promise to attend a ball game with Stu if one of our teams managed to make the playoffs. Since both of our teams were traditionally terrible, I figured it was a safe bet to make an old guy happy.

Then one day it was only Lynne in the lobby. She wasn't there for smores or RSO. She was there to tell me that her mother had passed, and that her father had followed his bride a very short time after. She gave me the kind of hug that would break your heart if you held on too long. She thanked me for helping her family and allowing Stu to be the only person that could get away with calling me a loser. With both of us laughing and crying, I made another promise, but this one to his daughter: that I would go to his funeral as requested. I had been working with medical marijuana patients for over ten years, and Stu's funeral still has been the only one I have attended. But, if having me at the funeral aided them in any way, I would be honored to help the family one last time.

To date, neither of our teams have made the playoffs since my promise to Stu. But when that day comes, I know it will be because Stu is pulling some strings upstairs for all us losers.

QUALITY OF LIFE

This means something different to all of us. For those that suffer with mental or emotional struggles, it can mean they make an active effort to protect their mental health, and these actions contribute to their quality of life. For those of us with physical limitations, this could mean a gadget, medicine, or way of thinking to just make our days a little bit less challenging. The Quality of Life Research Unit at the University of Toronto defines this as "how much a person can enjoy the valued possibilities of their lives."[122]

—

It was like any other Tuesday in a pot shop. An elderly woman, and what I assumed was her daughter, were standing on the opposite side of the counter from me, just like hundreds of others I have spoken with over the years. These conversations generally start with the younger of the two laying out their reasons for being there, while the older one looks around in a mix of awe, disbelief, and bashfulness. Let me tell you, Shirley was not impressed, and the farthest thing from bashful.

"You better not get me high! I'm not here to get high!" Shirley scolded. Trying not to feel like I was six years old being yelled at by Grandma, I reassured her that she did not have to get high to see if cannabis would be beneficial to her. I asked her the two most important questions in cannabis retail: "Have you spoken with your doctor about trying cannabis," and, "Do you take any prescriptions that have a grapefruit warning." After a satisfactory "yes," followed by a "no," we got into the reason she was standing before me.

Like so many others—too many others—Shirley's knowledge of cannabis came from a know-it-all neighbor, and a shoulder shrug from her doctor. She got her hands on someone's homemade topical, beginning to apply it once a week to her shoulder in hopes that it would replace the Percocet she had been saddled with for almost 30 years.

To this day I'm pretty sure my face spoke before my mouth did.

No wonder this feisty woman was in so much pain! Shirley stopped taking her prescribed painkiller of 30 years cold turkey. Trying to diminish my "bless your

---

[122] https://www.ncbi.nlm.nih.gov/books/NBK536962/

---

heart" tone of voice, I asked her how long ago she stopped taking the script, because Percocet does, in fact, come with a grapefruit warning. I wasn't so concerned about the topical usage and the drug interaction as I was about making a cannabis consumption recommendation of any kind with this painkiller in the mix. Shirley said it had been three months and she was very, very adamant about never taking it again.

This part of any cannabis consultation is always difficult if you're in it to help the patient. At some point you have to take the patient's word for it. These are adults and ultimately must be treated as such.

So, I let Shirley know how very important it was not to mix certain medications with cannabis as, depending on the drug, they could either make those drugs more or less potent. With a dismissive wave of her hand and a nod of acceptance, I explained why the topical wasn't touching her pain and took her through her possible choices. My go-to is always a low dose of CBD with new-to-cannabis patients, even those with the potential to have a tolerance due to long-term use of other medications. In this case it was a sugar-free hard candy. After all, what seasoned lady doesn't like hard candy? Before the package even hit the counter for her inspection, Shirley muttered under her breath that she better not get high.

Not wanting her to be distracted by this fear and have her actually learn about the plant and the products, I decided to fight moxy with moxy. "I'll tell you what, you can take me out into the intersection and kick my ass if I do sell you something that gets you high. BUT only if you promise to come back and let me know if it helps. AND you must take the product as suggested. You can't eat the whole bag of candy and then come in fists flying because you got high. Deal?" She agreed, made her purchase, grabbed her daughter (who had not gotten a single word in), and left me smiling the rest of the day. I love feisty women.

Shirley held up her end of the bargain and came back a few times to tweak the dosage and ratio, and to make my day. The last time I saw Shirley, she proudly told me that she finally bought eggs and milk again. Confused, I asked her if she had been boycotting cows and chickens, as plucky women have a tendency to do. Shaking her silver curls she said, "The pain got really bad there for a while, and I was so tired after grocery shopping that once I got home, I didn't have the strength to put the groceries away. I had to stop buying eggs and milk because they would spoil by the time I could recoup and unload the trunk."

———

I was punched in the heart that afternoon. I couldn't swallow the instant lump in my throat, all I could do was nod and keep watery eye contact. She stood taller as she said, "But today, Angie, I was able to put eggs and milk in my fridge again! Right after shopping! Can you believe it?!" Trying to make light of this very heavy statement and regain my composure, I said "Shirley! That's really fantastic news! And in more good news, I managed to avoid getting my ass kicked in public!" With a chuckle and twin smiles between us, Shirley made her purchase with confidence and went home to bake cupcakes for her grandkids from scratch for the first time in a long time.

DRUG ADDICTION

There are no two ways about it. Drug addiction is a very, very real concern, and should be treated as such. Addiction is diabolical and devastating to both the individual, and their loved ones. By definition, "Addiction is a treatable, chronic medical disease involving complex interactions among brain circuits, genetics, the environment, and an individual's life experiences."[123]

Addiction comes with many different moving parts, and make no mistake, cannabis is a drug. It comes with side effects (both good and bad), drug interactions, and legality issues. Over-education and open dialog with your doctors about your interest in cannabis is crucial.

Addiction is not only limited to "street drugs." Humans can be addicted to all sorts of things. Coffee, sugar, and the coveted runner's high are examples of common addictions. The jury is still out on why we take things, or why we do things that we know are bad for us. But what I do know is that when a person is willing to change their habits to better their health—to better their life—it is no small challenge, and they need an overabundance of compassion and guidance.

———

When I first met Gus, I can honestly say that I was afraid of him. He looked exactly like a junkie would look. Unbathed, grubby clothing, and a mouthful of

---

[123]https://www.asam.org/quality-care/definition-of-addiction

---

rotten teeth that looked like they would be evicted if he sneezed. He had a prominent limp, and his speech was slurred when he asked me for "strong smokes." Not really sure what he was asking for, and not wanting to have a conversation with his hot breath, I just pointed to the rows of flower on the opposite counter. Shaking his greasy mop feverishly, he responded with one word, "morphine." This got the attention of the door guy, and he moved in a bit closer to hear the exchange. "Morphine," he said again as he scratched his scabbed arms with intention. I sheepishly explained that we don't carry those kinds of drugs. "Good. Good. I don't want drugs. No more. No more morphine."

It turned out that Gus was looking to kick his morphine addiction with cannabis, and knew flower was not going to get the job done. I admittedly felt a bit better about the man swaying in front of me, put my faith into the hope that he wasn't there to do us any harm, and nodded the door guy back to his post. Still keeping my distance from the stench on this man and the potential of violence, I explained what might help with the withdrawals he was suffering at night and what may work for his daytime "strong smokes."

I knew enough about addiction that physical, chemical dependency is only half of the problem. Rituals and habits were the other half, and needed to be addressed if Gus was going to be successful. I remember being surprised when he pulled out enough cash to set him up for a month. I still use this memory to shame myself about wearing the white wig of judgment towards the outward appearance of others.

———

I honestly didn't think I'd see Gus again. I wanted him to succeed, but I've seen enough junkies that had the best of intentions and failed, nonetheless. I'm glad this guy proved me wrong. He came in a month later, and if it wasn't for the staggering limp, I wouldn't have known who he was. The physical change was so severe that I almost forgot how scared I was of this human in front of me just one month prior. Gus looked like he was cleaning up nicely, and flashed his new set of chompers as often as he could. He told me that he was now in the right frame of mind to tell me his unfortunate story. He had been smashed and mangled from a motorcycle accident. He had broken both hips and his pelvic bone in the crash, and once released from the hospital, the people at the rehab facility kept pumping an endless supply of morphine into his system. After leaving this last insurance-covered treatment, they wrote him an open-ended script for morphine in pill form.

I had never heard of such a thing! It has always been my opinion that if you are in such rough shape that you need heavy hitters such as morphine or fentanyl, your ass should still be in the hospital under the strict eye of the doctor doing the prescribing. Alas, this is not how the world works, and it wasn't a surprise that Gus ended up with a very serious addiction.

———

The good news here is that Gus was a fighter and was not about to give up on his young life. As he was more able to come into the shop, we worked together to begin bringing down his cannabis dosage. I won't lie, there were some setbacks, and a lot of trial and error, but the day did come when the only purchase Gus made was for a couple of pre-rolls for a road trip with his old riding crew.

ANXIETY

As defined by the American Psychological Association, "Anxiety is an emotion characterized by feelings of tension, worried thoughts, and physical changes like increased blood pressure. People with anxiety disorders usually have recurring intrusive thoughts or concerns. They may avoid certain situations out of worry. They may also have physical symptoms such as sweating, trembling, dizziness, or a rapid heartbeat."

In today's crazy world, anxiety triggers are everywhere. A busy parking lot, an overcrowded lobby, and the stress of communicating with a stranger in a chaotic environment can sometimes be overstimulating for anyone. And since people with anxiety have their own ways of coping with it, it can sometimes be difficult to recognize it as a medical condition, instead of just some random weirdo.

———

We had a woman that had made several attempts to purchase cannabis from us. The first time I noticed her was on a very busy Wednesday, where she walked in, took one look around, and left. I just chalked it up to her not wanting to wait. The next day she made it to the receptionist but bolted before her name was

---

[124]*https://www.apa.org/topics/anxiety/*

---

called. Two days later she made it until her name was called and was escorted to a budtender for a consultation. She asked about edibles, and when her budtender asked if she preferred candy or baked goods, she made a 180 degree turn and ran for the door. Of course, at this point I asked the consultant what the deal was, which was answered by a shoulder shrug and a "dunno." I pulled her name up in the system and added a note saying, "may have anxiety about small or noisy spaces. If available, have Angie consult."

———

If memory serves, it was only a few hours later when the woman tried again, and I was called to the counter. I didn't want to freak her out by asking about her behavior or let on that I had asked about the issue just a few hours prior. You could tell this woman was very uncomfortable, but wanted nothing more than to finally get what she came for on her third attempt.

I took her to the station at the far end of the room to get as much privacy as was possible in the small space. Direct eye contact seemed to make her more nervous, so I pretended to be busy picking at a sticker on the counter while I asked her questions. Just as I was starting to feel pretty good about my approach with the woman, she whispered "I'm sorry. I can't," and hightailed it out of the building. Out of ideas, I set aside the items I had talked about and set them aside with her name on it.

About 15 minutes prior to closing, the woman was in our med room for the fourth time that day. I once again took the consultation on myself, headed to the same station, and grabbed her bag that I had set aside. She looked at me with both appreciation and embarrassment. Before she could speak, I let her know that in fact, we had a couple of employees that suffered from anxiety, and when busy, the circus that was a pot shop in those days could be very overwhelming to the best of us.

I then took the small window of opportunity to offer that we did offer online ordering where she could browse our menu, place an order, and it would be made ready for her to pick up from reception (curbside wasn't a thing yet). I also made sure she had my number in case she had any questions or concerns. As it turned out, this woman placed online orders every Friday like clockwork, which made me happy knowing that she was getting the medicine she needed without having to stir up her affliction.

ALZHEIMER'S

According to the Mayo Clinic, "Alzheimer's disease is a progressive neurologic disorder that causes the brain to shrink (atrophy) and brain cells to die. Alzheimer's disease is the most common cause of dementia—a continuous decline in thinking, behavioral and social skills that affects a person's ability to function independently.

Approximately 5.8 million people in the United States age 65 and older live with Alzheimer's disease. Of those, 80% are 75 years old and older. Out of the approximately 50 million people worldwide with dementia, between 60% and 70% are estimated to have Alzheimer's disease."[125]

Not everyone takes the same approach as I do when it comes to educating cannabis retail staff. I'm more of a "Go ahead ... touch the stove. Was it hot? Will you do it again?" kind of teacher. And I always knew which regular patients to use for my lessons with new hires to get my point across.

—

Marvin was the living, breathing human version of Mr. Magoo. As you can imagine it took the patience of a saint to help this gentleman with his purchases, and therefore, he was unknowingly a part of my training process.

Scott, a new hire, was fitting in nicely, but the opportunity still hadn't presented itself yet to see how he handled an Alzheimer patient. The rest of the staff knew Marvin pretty well at this point and knew exactly what I was doing when I told reception to make sure that he was helped by Scott that morning.

Being naturally kind, Scott introduced himself with a smile while looking into Marvin's notes for guidance in his consultation. Marvin was naturally opposed to change, and tested Scott on his past purchases after pointing out that he was new. I busied myself with organizing inventory within earshot of the conversation to judge how much of Marvin Scott could take before his patience slipped.

Thirty minutes went by, and Scott was finally cashing Marvin out. All and all, the new guy did a fantastic job throughout the whole transaction. He even stayed friendly when Marvin asked to see the same package four different times.

And then Scott slipped.

---

[125] https://www.mayoclinic.org/diseases-conditions/alzheimers-disease/symptoms-causes/syc-20350447

Marvin was struggling with counting out the change he had in the palm of his hand. Coke bottles for eyeglasses or not, anyone could see that he couldn't see. This had been the subject of many conversations around the reception desk because the thought of this guy getting behind the wheel terrified us all. We also knew that this was the longest part of helping Marvin.

He would hold up each coin and turn it around in the light, double checking that the coin was in fact what he thought it was, before placing it in the pile on the glass top with the others. As Marvin held up another coin, Scott let go of a heavy sigh and said, "yep ... that's a nickel," in such a way that I couldn't help but to laugh. It was like laughing in church. It made it that much more entertaining because you weren't supposed to laugh. I hightailed it to my office in the back to regain my composure.

Another 20 minutes went by before Scott came into the back, marking the end of his first consultation with Marvin. I applauded him for his patience, apologized for my lack of giggle control, and I rewarded him with a 15-minute break.

CHRONIC PAIN

According to the Cleveland Clinic, "Chronic pain is a very common condition, and one of the most common reasons why someone seeks medical care. Approximately 25% of adults in the United States experience chronic pain. Chronic pain is pain that lasts for over three months. The pain can be there all the time, or it may come and go. It can happen anywhere in your body. Chronic pain can interfere with your daily activities, such as working, having a social life and taking care of yourself or others. It can lead to depression, anxiety and trouble sleeping, which can make your pain worse."[126]

Chronic pain is also the most common category for those seeking relief through cannabis. Such a blanketed term can cover anything from headaches to ALS. This type of relentless pain not only affects you physically, but emotionally and mentally as well. The National Library of Medicine published the following opinion of Dac Teoli and Abhishek Bhardwaj, which urge medical professionals to treat not just the problem, but the person. "All interprofessional healthcare team members, including clinicians, mid-level practitioners, specialists, nurses, pharma-

---

[126]https://www.mayoclinic.org/diseases-conditions/alzheimers-disease/symptoms-causes/syc-20350447

---

cists, mental health professionals, therapists, and other ancillary healthcare personnel, need to recognize the concept of quality of life. It is crucial to remember that the team is treating a person, not just a set of lab values or pathology, and treatment goals need to keep the patient's QOL in mind and focus toward that outcome in conjunction with addressing medical needs."[127]

Please and Thank You

As you can imagine, I have told my own personal cannabis story more than once, and to more than one audience. Sometimes I tell it to give the positive side of cannabis a human face, and other times I tell it to gain trust and credibility with patients that don't seem quite convinced about my experience with pain.

Charcot Marie Tooth (CMT) has run rampant throughout my family for generations now. It's a neurodegenerative disease that affects 1 in 2500 people in the United States and 2.6 million worldwide (last I checked), making this the most common hereditary disease out there, yet it is considered a "rare" disease. Go figure. And because it is misdiagnosed more times than not, the numbers are thought to be much higher than reported. CMT causes muscle wasting, deformities in the feet and hands, and the gait of a stork (imaging walking in scuba flippers); it comes with the frigid numbness or random blow torch-like bee stings that are included with nerve damage, and all kinds of embarrassing balance issues. I could be standing in line at the grocery store and WHAM, I'm stumbling two steps to the left and one step back, just trying not to fall down in public. Some of the muscles in my hands are long gone, which makes anything that requires dexterity a joke, and because braces have never worked for me, I can only effectively walk in high, laced-up boots (never comfortable when on an island vacation).

I won't lie, it's not great. There is no cure. But I will say that it's pretty rare for me to be in bedridden pain, and the disease won't kill me, it's just a real pain in my ass to live with. The words of Caddyshack's Carl Spackler, "So I got that going for me, which is nice," perfectly sums up my efforts to remain positive.

---

[127] https://www.ncbi.nlm.nih.gov/books/NBK536962/

In my mid-30s I was a working realtor, a single mom, and I was taking mountains of pills at every meal for more than one reason. Some were for pain, some were beta blockers, and some were to combat the side effects of all the other prescriptions. Then I began having kidney issues. By issues, I mean I was passing kidney stones every few weeks, and when I couldn't pass them on my own, I would find myself in the hospital for days on end.

So, at my next neurologist appointment (where I was getting all these prescriptions), I asked her why. Without looking up from the chart in her hand, she said, "It's to be expected, and will only get worse as you age. You've been taking pills for so long that your kidneys were bound to have issues eventually. I can start you on a medication that should help with kidney stones." A switch flipped in my brain. What? Really? Yet another drug to clean up after the other drugs I was already taking?

"I'm going to pass," I said with a voice I had forgotten I had. "Adding another pill to the mix doesn't seem like it would be helping the situation any. I'm going to look into it myself and see if there is a different way to fix this." Clearly exhausted by my desire to have a conversation, she responded with, "Suit yourself. Don't forget to set your next appointment on the way out," and she walked out of the room.

———

For the first time in my life, I felt like I had some sort of say in my healthcare. That I had some sort of control over the piles of pills I consumed daily. I pushed past my vintage frustrations with my doctors and focused on this new self-made path. The question at that moment was: now what do I do with that control?

I had heard that more and more people were getting state-issued medical marijuana cards in Michigan for certain disabilities. Keep in mind that the only weed that I had had up to this point was the stuff that circulated around high school parking lots and 4th of July bonfires. I honestly did not believe at the time that marijuana was going to fix my kidney issues, but what did I have to lose at this point besides face?

So, I found a certification doctor that was local enough and reasonable enough, cost wise, to set an appointment. Some of these places would charge up to $500, and therefore were too expensive for a single mom's bank account.

The day had finally arrived, and as I waited among dozens of people, all with the hopes that they would get the okay from the doctor to begin helping themselves with cannabis, it dawned on me that I couldn't grow. In fact, many a cactus had died by my hands in my attempts to grow something—anything. You know those dancing solar flowers? Yeah, those stop when I walk into the room. It's an utter miracle that my kid not only survived but thrived under my care.

—

With this fresh anxiety I looked around the room for anyone who appeared like they could give me some direction. On my left was an elderly woman that looked friendly enough to put my delicate question to. "Excuse me ma'am. Can I ask where you get your marijuana from?" The word "cannabis" wasn't second nature yet, and it still didn't sit with me that it should be referred to as "medicine." The woman pulled her purse closer to her chest, and in the exact opposite manner to her physical reaction, she began to give up the goods like she was elated that someone had finally asked.

"Your first card, honey?" she asked, but didn't give the time for an answer.

"I've had mine since the beginning. I put it on everything. You know you can make butter with it, don't you dear? It's easy. Stinky, but easy. Just a slow cooker and some cheese cloth. I put it on everything. Did I already say that? Oops. Well, I do. I put it on my toast in the morning and it's really good with fish and all kinds of other things I like to eat." I was shocked and delighted all at once. This old lady was on top of it! I was about to reiterate my initial question when the guy on my right tapped my knee and whispered, "I can help."

I immediately felt like we were breaking the law just for having this conversation. It turned out that we knew some of the same people from the area, and he was in fact a registered caregiver with the state. He was there with a patient of his to renew her card, and he offered me the last patient spot he had open (in Michigan you are allowed five). I responded with gratitude and tucked his number safely away.

Once the paperwork for making him my caregiver came back from the state, we had a long conversation about what my expectations were for both him and cannabis. I explained the situation, and upon mentioning the number of pharmaceuticals I was taking, he confidently said, "We have some work to do, but I think cannabis can help."

Over the next year or so I successfully weaned myself off of all of my prescriptions. I started with taking a dose of FECO instead of taking a Norco, and from there slowly began substituting cannabis for all of my medications. In my opinion, the beta blockers were the worst to kick. I'm still unsure if it was because I had been taking those the longest, or if it had something to do with the stranglehold they held over my system. It wasn't pretty, and I wasn't a nice person during this, but I did it.

I would never, ever recommend anyone stop taking their doctor-prescribed medication. This course of action was how I chose to handle it, and in hindsight, it would've probably been easier on me (and my family) if I had a doctor to work with in stepping down these medications.

Once free from the persecution of prescriptions, I set an appointment with the same neurologist that was my former dealer. We moved through the balance tests and pin pricks that are standard with these types of appointments and got into what scripts I needed refilled. "None," I answered proudly. This got her to actually look up from the chart and into my eyes. "I don't need a damn one of them filled, thank you very much. I haven't taken any of them for months now and don't plan on taking them ever again." I thought she would be at the very least intrigued. Nope.

"You can't just stop taking what I have told you to take. The withdrawals can be very harmful and are only to be done with my consent and under my care." To this day I'm still not sure how the doctor, her ego, and myself all fit in the same small exam room.

"Too late. Over a year ago you told me that I should expect kidney problems, that they would only get worse, and to just take another pill as my health deteriorated. I found this to be unacceptable. So, I decided to try cannabis as medicine. It worked. It's still working. And you know what? I haven't had a kidney stone in over nine months now," I informed her as I climbed off the table and reached for my coat.

"It will stop working. You'll be back." It has been almost 13 years since this conversation, and I have zero intentions of returning to the woman.

Please understand me. I'm not saying that I don't need doctors. I'm not saying that I don't need a neurologist to monitor the progression of my disease. What I'm saying here is that a doctor has the responsibility to "do no harm," and through my experiences to date, I would say too many have either forgotten this, or just straight up disregard it. Upon hearing of my kidney issues, this doctor should have first put down the chart and looked at me. Second, she should've pulled up my list of scripts to see what I could do without to lessen the burden on my organs. Should'a, could'a, would'a.

My current doctors know exactly how to treat me, because they know that cannabis is always my first choice in medication. But if cannabis isn't cutting it and I am sitting in front of them, freezing my ass off in a paper towel dress, they know it's because I need them to work with me, not against me.

VETERANS

Our government entity of Veterans Affairs (VA) can be taxing, to say the very least, when it comes to helping our military. There is a lack of modernized care, benefits are given and then taken away, pills are overprescribed, and the suicide rate is at atrocious levels.

According to the USO, "In 2021, research found that 30,177 active-duty personnel and veterans who served in the military after 9/11 have died by suicide—compared to the 7,057 service members killed in combat in those same 20 years. That is, military suicide rates are four times higher than deaths that occurred during military operations."[128]

With the VA policies being too stubborn to evolve, you can imagine the battle our service members have to fight to get any alternative therapies accepted. So, for a boots-on-the-ground report, I reached out to my old friend Domingo. In the following sentences, he will tell the story about what it is truly like to be a US veteran fighting the system when it comes to his healthcare.

---

[128]https://www.uso.org/stories/2664-military-suicide-rates-are-at-an-all-time-high-heres-how-were-trying-to-help

Domingo and I met working at a shop over a decade ago. He, like so many other veterans, had turned to cannabis as a method of treatment in order to fill the huge gaps that the VA healthcare wasn't covering.

Domingo signed up as a healthy young American and was a hospital corpsman during his two-year enlistment in the US Navy, tacking on another year in the reserves. By the end of his three years, he had picked up an ugly collection of PTSD, alcoholism, autoimmune dysfunction, Pancolitis, hidradenitis suppurativa, and insomnia. He tells me that he has no doubt that these medical conditions were due to his time spent with the Navy.

I had asked him what his first VA visit was like once returning home. "My first experience with the VA was a year or two after I left active service. I was required by Veterans Treatment Court to meet with a therapist for PTSD. The therapist dismissed my military trauma and was rude/indifferent to my plight. They prescribed me multiple antidepressants, which made things worse. I never went back to them." And when asked if he saw any difference between the VA and "regular" healthcare, Domingo said, "Not really, both community-based clinics and VA hospitals are constrained by the same bureaucracy. Obviously, hospitals are bigger, have more departments, and are a little cleaner; but both of them practice medicine one dimensionally."

I had asked him to explain what it was like to ask for alternative therapies from a government-run medical facility, and if he has seen any changes in the last ten years. I asked for these details because I want to give my readers a bird's eye view of what can be realistically expected for other veterans. This is how he explains it.

———

"My first discussion for alternative therapies was about cannabis for my ulcerative colitis. VA doctors (even the one alternative healthcare-certified physician that I see) have maintained it has no medicinal value; it is a Schedule I narcotic and so it's highly addictive, and that 'we all will probably look back at legalization and regret it.'

"Being a cannabis user under the VA's care has made it difficult for the doctors to prescribe pain meds for when I'm in serious pain; it's also resulted in being flagged in their system as an 'illegal drug abuser,' which affects how they treat/view me as a person."

Domingo went on to say, "My VA care has been the same for the last decade: treating symptoms with 'evidence-based medicine' (big pharma funded data) without knowing root causes. No known root cause = no known cure. The policy on medical cannabis supposedly changed from being 'a no go,' to docs being able to talk to their patients about it (just talk). Based on my conversations with an array of specialists, it's still a no go."

———

In 2017, the VA addressed the can's and cannot's of veterans using cannabis as medicine. But the VA cannot recommend, fill out paperwork, or pay for a veteran's cannabis. And as Domingo harshly found out, those in white coats at the VA are still extremely prejudiced against the plant, and the patients using it.[129]

I asked Domingo what advice he could give to other veterans who struggle with these frustrations when it comes to the care that is provided for them from the VA's iron-fisted standard procedures and protocols.

"Do what works for you. The VA is one dimensional and will close you off to treatments outside their purview. In our healing journey, we must remain open to ALL available remedies. Just because the VA isn't, doesn't mean you have to be. Consider alternative medicine, and depending on your medical situation, you may be able to just take that route. For some of us, we will have to negotiate between the two systems, and that's OK too.

"Advocate for your values and yourself because NO one else will; your VA healthcare team won't, your patient advocate won't, your local political representatives won't. All they will do is make sure the VA is following its own standard operating procedure. So, work the system, because all it seems to offer is a gloomy outlook of inevitable decrepitude (your diseases have no known root cause or cure and are progressive in their nature) that's made "tolerable" with pharmaceuticals.

"But don't just survive ... try to thrive! Go outside the VA. Find people and organizations that support your healing journey and seek those who won't close you off to treatments that could change your quality of life for the better."

In wrapping up the interview, I asked Domingo to recommend any veterans groups that he has found to be honest and helpful in our cannabis war at home.

---

[129]https://www.publichealth.va.gov/marijuana.asp

They are the following: Fallen Wounded Soldiers, Concerned Veterans of America, Balanced Veterans Network, Operation 1620, Project Triangle, and the Veterans Cannabis Project.

—

I thought about putting the following personal story under a PTSD section of this book. Then I said to myself, "Self, PTSD is a problem, not a person." Not all veterans have PTSD, and not all PTSD comes from war zones. For me, being in the medical cannabis space is about helping the entire human, not just their afflictions.

I am a big college football fan (Go Blue) and try to watch as many games as I can. This season while enjoying the Army vs. Navy game, the announcer said something that rekindled my feelings about our veterans. The announcer said, "Every single team member on either side of the ball is willing to die for you." It's not that I didn't already know this very heavy statement, it was just a gentle reminder to me how committed our military truly is, active duty or not.

In my time on this rock, I have known a few military men, and it wasn't just because of the uniforms (okay, maybe a couple of times). I have a sincere sweet spot for our military and their families, because I know what it is like to live with loved ones who suffer from the aftereffects that this type of service can cause.

—

On a busy day where nobody seemed to want to return on time after lunch, I ended up at a station moving patients along. A mountain of a man came through the door, and I found myself not breathing. Maybe for others it was his six foot seven, 320-pound (if he was a day), attention-grabbing frame, but for me it was the vapor of pure frustration and simmering rage that came off of this man like a fever. I would love to tell you that this was an educated assessment, instead of the sour truth of knowing this particular fever from a very personal trauma. It was quite different from the hysteria you can feel from tweaking drug addicts, which was mostly urgency and disdain. Whether this disgust was for the human race or themselves, I cannot say. But this guy had the slow boil of anger that came back with veterans that had breathed and bathed in war.

I quickly scanned the room for Jones, the only veteran we had on staff that day, for two reasons. First, I was beginning to lose my cool, and second because

I knew no one could help this man better than a fellow brother in arms. But to my dismay, our on-site corpsman had just settled into what is usually a lengthy consult with a regular patient. When I caught his eye at the far end of the room, I could see that he was definitely paying attention to my interaction with the giant. He could feel the fever too. But unable to get away from his own consultation, he could only keep one watchful eye on me.

Momentarily dazed from the brutish push down memory lane, I found him standing directly before me. Do you remember the Bugs Bunny cartoons when a huge, heavy-breathing hulk of a man would loom over him? It was like that. I stand tall at a grand five foot nothing, so yeah, it was exactly like that.

Military members are almost always attracted to the "rush" sativa terpenes offer, and therefore I pulled all of the heavy zingers off the shelf for his inspection. I fumbled through the remainder of the consultation, finding myself on the same eggshells of my yesterdays. He eventually chose the third offering with a grunt, while I tried to still my shaking hands.

Honestly, in hindsight, he wasn't rude or loud or challenging in any way. This one was totally on me. I was stunned that I had such an uncharacteristic emotional reaction to this guy who was only there wanting help. I harshly reminded myself that people like this is one of the reasons why I'm in the cannabis industry in the first place, and then scolded myself for losing focus.

Once past this mental self-therapy, I tried to extend the conversation after the sale as a last-ditch effort to help him. I asked about sleeping habits, what he does with his days, and whether he was in touch with the VA. Of course, the last question stirred him up, and out the door he went.

I did see him again and was grateful that I didn't botch it badly enough to keep him from coming back. I also found myself holding my breath again. Apparently, it takes more than one self-therapy session to mop up the mud.

This time he got himself to the nearest station (thankfully it was Jones') and began to speak to me over the tops of the heads in the room a few stations down. Giving him the hold-on-a-minute hand signal, I made my way over to him to keep him from shouting across the room. Admittedly, I felt a bit better about the situation this time around knowing that my corpsman would be right there if I should need any assistance (personally or otherwise).

I wasn't next to Jones for ten seconds when this guy leans his tree trunk of a torso over the counter and wraps me up in a hug. I'm pretty sure I blacked out, and I am nowhere near composure when he lets go and returns his upper half to its original position. "Thank you. It was hard for me being here last time. You were nice to me. Thank you." he said with a lower voice. I could've wept for both him and I right there, but all I could muster was the canned response of "Happy to help." I nodded to Jones in gratitude for his loyalty and as I walked away, I heard Jones tell the man, "I got you brother." Indeed, I thought. You might be the only one that does.

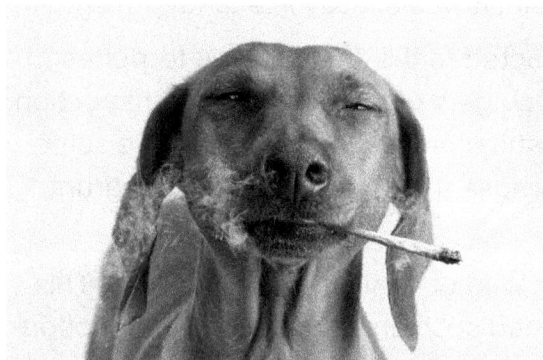

PETS

We all love our fur babies and would do pretty much anything to ease any of their suffering. All animals have an endocannabinoid system, just as we do, but the difference is that our pets break down and distribute cannabinoids differently.

Dogs don't do great with consuming THC. Whether they are given this intoxicating compound intentionally, or they got into your stash, it can put your pooch in a bad way. They are prone to "static ataxia," which is defined by the medical dictionary as "a loss of deep sensibility, causing the inability to preserve equilibrium in standing."[130] In English, this means they will stumble around, or may even be unable to get themselves up on their own four paws, much like a drunken sailor, with doses of THC as low as 0.5 mgs.[131] Yet studies are showing that your pets can safely tolerate much higher levels of CBD. These studies also bring attention to the oils that these cannabinoids are offered in, as they are often the culprit for any stomach distress.[132]

130https://medical-dictionary.thefreedictionary.com/static+ataxia
131https://www.ncbi.nlm.nih.gov/pmc/articles/PMC6770351/

If you believe that Fido has gotten into your edibles, the following signs may be used to confirm whether you should get him to the vet ASAP.

THE MOST COMMON SIGNS OF EXCESS CANNABIS EXPOSURE IN DOGS AND CATS[133]

NEUROLOGICAL
- Sleepiness
- Ataxia

DEPRESSION
- Wobbling, pacing and agitation
- Vocalization

EYES
- Dilated pupils
- Bloodshot eyes

GASTRO-INTESTINAL
- Vomiting
- Salivation

OTHERS
- Sound or light sensitivity
- Inappropriate urination

FAST OR SLOW HEART RATES
- Low body temperature

[132]https://pubmed.ncbi.nlm.nih.gov/32118071/

[133]De Briyne N, Holmes D, Sandler I, Stiles E, Szymanski D, Moody S, Neumann S, Anadón A. Cannabis, Cannabidiol Oils and Tetrahydrocannabinol-What Do Veterinarians Need to Know? Animals (Basel). 2021 Mar 20;11(3):892. doi: 10.3390/ani11030892. PMID: 33804793; PMCID: PMC8003882.

POLICY

"What a way to run a railroad."
– Bugs Bunny

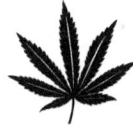

DISCLAIMER

The following policy experiences and opinions come from my work in the medical cannabis retail arena. But these lessons and suggestions can and absolutely should be applied to adult-use businesses. Some states have had hundreds of thousands of medical cannabis patients prior to opening up with adult use. Reports from all over the country will show you how the medical card holder numbers fall through the floor once rec passes. But it's not like all of the med patients just ceased to exist. There are still those massive groups, it's just that they prefer not to be on "the list" when it comes to their cannabis consumption. So, even if your location and/or products are deemed "recreational" or "adult use," keep in mind that all cannabis is medicinal.

I also want to address those that do not work in the cannabis industry who will read the following section on policy. If I had to guess, I'd say most of you have worked in some sort of retail, customer service, or hospitality position in your lives. You get it. You understand that it's hard work. You understand that the person behind the counter is only there to help you. You also know that humans can be complete jerks sometimes. This is very much a daily truth in the cannabis retail space. The following policy stories and recommendations are almost wholly from humans behaving badly, on both sides of the counter.

But make no mistake, I loved my time in cannabis retail! Yes, the hours were long, and the work was physically and mentally challenging. But no two days were the same, I adored my co-workers, and I was always learning something new. There isn't quite anything like the rush of looking around the store under your control and seeing that the place is packed, knowing your staff is an intelligent, well-oiled rig, and that people are happy.

———

I have learned, sometimes painfully, that you simply cannot be prepared for every situation that walks into a pot shop. Humans are still so widely unpredictable that even after more than a decade of working behind the cannabis retail counter, I was still surprised almost every day. One of the best things you can do for your company, your staff, and yourself, is to pay attention and learn from the "Well, that sucked. Let's not have that happen again," events. Change that expensive standard operating procedure. Modify that membership agreement. Listen, I mean seriously listen to the employees that are on the frontlines of your business.

As the saying goes, "Adapt or die."

PRODUCT KNOWLEDGE

I know brands out there will argue, after all they have spent heavy coin to get in front of the consumer, but to be successful you should above all want to be helpful. It has been said that in sales you should "sell the problem it solves, not the product." This is beyond true in the cannabis space.

Getting to know the products you carry inside and out will not only help your patients, but also increase the cannabis intelligence of your budtenders. Make no mistake, your patients are paying attention. They know that the orange ABC gummies tested out higher this time around than the cherry. Do you? Every time a new order comes in the door, check out the test results specific to that batch. You may have been ordering this brand for months, but each batch can vary.

Cannabinoid content is just as important as the manufacturing process (e.g. is it distillate or whole plant) and so is the integrity of the company behind the brand.

So many of us choose sides every day. Some refuse to shop at certain grocery stores because of the treatment of their staff, while others will boycott another retailer due to their political beliefs. So why shouldn't it be the same in cannabis? Is it because some brands and their dirty laundry are not plastered all over the evening news? Or is it because to buy marijuana legally is still a novel privilege and some people just want their product to be cheap and effective? I'd say it's a little column A and a little column B.

I say we take "branding" out of the conversation. If your product is really the cat's pajamas, it won't need flashy packaging or celebrity endorsements. Budtenders everywhere will always push what works for them, regardless of the fancy swag you dole out on vender days.

Once we had a vendor day with a company that quite honestly had a garbage product. They came with bright banners, a buy three get the fourth for free enticement, and even vape batteries engraved with each budtenders name. Yes, it brought in a slightly bigger crowd, but the staff knew better. Their carts were famous for leaking, containing heavy cutting agents, and always tasted like perfume. Not a single budtender bought the carts to go with their newly monogrammed batteries.

MANAGING YOUR PHYSICAL SPACE

Not everyone has the opportunity to build their retail location from scratch. The majority have to take what they can get given strict zoning issues, regardless of what state you are in. Out of the five dispensaries that I have worked at, a few were old houses converted into a commercial space and came with some challenges regarding the functionality.

These converted homes had steep steps leading to the front door and suck-in-your-gut narrow doorways once inside. At one place the door guy, and whatever strong staff member they could find, would have to carry the patient's wheelchair up the stairs and squeeze it through the doorway. These patients and their chairs couldn't make it through the second doorway, which led to the med room. A budtender would have to run back and forth showing products to the patient. In another location they had a ramp out back, but once inside the patient found himself in the back inventory room and would have to navigate their way into the med room from behind the counter. This setup was completely against the law, as no one that was not an employee or approved vendor was allowed access to the area.

Now, how awful is this for the patient! The Americans with Disabilities Act is there for a reason folks. People with wheelchairs, walkers, crutches, and canes, have every right to be able to access store fronts, and not through the back door like third class citizens.

These obstacles can be overcome with some creative thinking. It can be as simple as putting a rug over a threshold for easier rolling and less of a tripping hazard. Or it can be as big as opening up a doorway, changing stairs into a ramp, or adding double handrails. Another way you can accommodate your customers is by keeping chairs and a wheelchair available for anyone who may need them. Cannabis compassion is more than just shoveling the snow from the walkway.

—

People in general really don't need much to profess their loyalty to a company. I have found that honesty and transparency will secure their homage. You really don't have to spend too much time or money on these efforts either. I have seen countless approaches to make yourself stand out from the rest in attempts to retain their customer base. Some were as novel as spinning a carnival wheel to see what percentage got knocked off their bill, to offering to roll a joint on the spot with any of the flower on the shelves. This one was a bit counterproductive to the patient flow, in my opinion. A budtender had to stop what they were doing, weigh out the gram, grind it up and hand roll the joint while others were waiting in line just to be seen. If you have ever worked in the restaurant business, I can compare this to someone asking for a hand-squeezed pitcher of lemonade during the dinner rush.

> **Tip:** Something I believe to be extra important is having a binder with all of the test results available for patients to review. If you (or your vendors) are not doing anything wrong, you have nothing to hide, right? Plus, this is a great way to educate the consumer on how your Purple Punch is pretty much the same thing as your Grape Stomper.

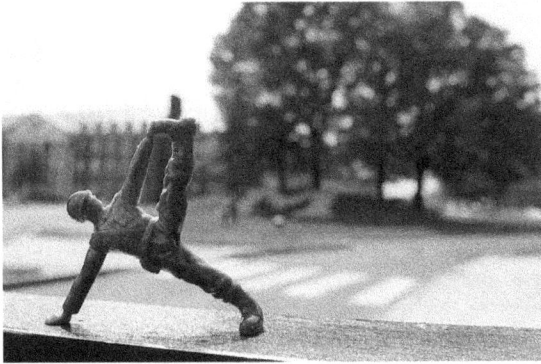

WHO TO HIRE
(WITH OR WITHOUT EXPERIENCE)

When staffing a retail cannabis establishment, recognize that you are, in fact, building an army. Your hires should include communications, intelligence, muscle, and of course, special forces.

———

Your hand-picked staff will be the boots on the ground of your retail operation. Understanding that not all situations can be successfully managed by traditional methods will be a major key to your success. Dealing with product refunds and state-sanctioned purchasing limits will require more than just good guidelines; you'll need staff with the skills to actually execute them in real time.

So, instead of hiring those that are only in it because it would be cool to sling weed, staff your business with your own medical condition specialists. One should be an ace in anxiety, another a devil dog of depression, and another a decorated captain of chronic pain, as these are the most common conditions that will cross your threshold.

———

Employees with first-hand knowledge of suffering from these conditions themselves, or having loved ones that do, will reinforce your reputation with your patients and strengthen the confidence in their care. These life-experienced personnel, when strategically placed, create your own unique synergy, your own entourage effect, if you will.

A consultant who suffers with anxiety themselves can confidently and honestly recommend what cannabis products work, or don't work, for them personally. These conversations, on a shared condition and with firsthand experiences, will create a bond of true understanding. The healing process for a patient seems a bit less daunting, a little less lonely, knowing that someone else has been where they are now. It is these kinds of connections that are a dispensary's biggest staffing asset in retaining patient loyalty.

At one point, I had worked with a fantastic consultant that had unfortunately been in a tragic car accident, which put her into a wheelchair. Her upbeat look at life, and visibly obvious personal knowledge of what it means to be in pain, had patients waiting in line to be specifically seen by her. They knew she could relate and was on top of the latest and greatest cannabis products available for relentless chronic pain.

Taking advice from someone who has never lived day in and day out with the mental struggles that come with physical pain, or the physical side effects from mental anguish, is like having a dietitian that doesn't care for cake. They can explain the textbook science behind why your body craves sweets, but that's where it ends. They can sympathize, but never really understand the place you are coming from.

———

I have also always believed having veterans in our ranks not only employs our honorable service men and women, but they also share an unspoken bond with others that have served. Whether it is—what seems like to most of us—coded language and inside jokes, or just a look and a nod, there is a healing comradery in the time they spend together. The fact that their service may have been decades and oceans apart has little bearing. The veterans on staff can recommend medication without verbally pushing a private veteran into dumping their emotional baggage out on the counter. These relations are worth their weight in gold. Not only to the establishment and its reputation, but more importantly, the wellbeing of the patient.

MINORS AND THEIR CAREGIVERS

There seems to be an all-out panic that runs through a shop when a minor is in the lobby. We have been so conditioned that cannabis is the devil's lettuce, and we must "save the children," that we forget that sometimes a child is in fact the patient.

Make no mistake, cannabis, in any form, should be locked up just like your liquor cabinet or your prescriptions for the safety of everyone involved. But when the proper steps have been taken by a parent to legally register their child as a medical marijuana patient, it is safe to say that they are only there as a last-ditch effort to help their kid.

———

When the regulated medical market started in Michigan, everyone was so skittish that they seemed to have forgotten the caregiver laws that had been in place since 2008. Under this law, in order for a minor to receive the blessings of the state for medical cannabis, they have to have two separate recommendations. One from their pediatrician and one from another doctor. A parent also must be tied to them as their caregiver. Assuming all of this was on the up and up, both the parent and the minor were allowed into marijuana retail shops. Yet the higher ups would become unglued when they saw these couples in the lobby. I have experienced this a few times, but the one that really sticks was one where I had to defend a young man that had the exact same rare disease that I do.

———

The receptionist called me to the front to double check on the legality of a mother and minor looking to come in, and after seeing that everything was in order, I allowed them into the med room. Not ten seconds later, one of the higher ups came flying into the room and made a beeline for me and the mother and son at the counter. "He can't be in here! He's clearly underage so we can't sell him anything. He HAS to go now!" Having been shamed, the mother and son began to move away from the counter to leave.

"Stop," I said with visible embarrassment for the ignorance of the boss. "Let me see your cards again," I asked the mom. Laying the cards next to each other on the counter for inspection, I replied, "Yep. Both cards are valid and unexpired.

Under our caregiver laws this young man is well within his rights to be in here as long as he is accompanied by his caregiver, which is this patient lady standing in front of you." Because he was made to look like the ass that he was, he snapped back with, "I'd feel a lot better if she left him in the car and just made the purchase herself." Mind you this was a sixteen-year-old boy that he was treating like a toddler.

"Why shouldn't this young man be allowed to learn about the medicine he's taking? Do you have any idea how useful this information would have been for me when I was young? He needs to know this stuff for when he turns eighteen and starts going to these places by himself," I clapped back. Not another word came out of the higher up's mouth as he slinked away from the unnecessary altercation with his ego tucked between his legs.

I apologized to both of them for the interruption and continued with the consultation. Learning that the teenager had the exact same disability that I did really helped with my recommendations (and warnings), and today I still feel like I did my job to the fullest extent, my superiors be damned. I not only stood up for the duo, but I also gave them a sounding board that made them feel we knew what they were going through.

COVERING YOUR BASES WHEN CATERING TO PATIENTS

Some retail locations are placed to cater to assisted living facilities in the area. I worked in one such location where it was common that residents would use their motorized scooters to come by for their medication. They would leave their transportation on the back stoop where they could plug it in for a quick charge while they were shopping. It seemed to work pretty well for everyone involved, until it didn't.

—

Hank came to see us every Thursday and knew the routine. What he failed to mention is that his scooter had been on the fritz and was struggling to hold a charge. So even though we had plugged in his ride, the thing wouldn't start when he had finished shopping. I wasn't really sure how to handle the situation with Hank in my wheeled office chair and his dead horse. After being informed that there wasn't anyone to come to get him, as his housing complex didn't run shuttles on Thursdays, I called him an Uber on my dime. While we waited, I tried to get in touch with the facility to let them know that we had his scooter and that we could keep it overnight, if need be, but that was the absolute extent that we could keep it in the shop. My call was not met with much concern for Hank and his horse, only a "We'll see what we can do." Though this response was not helpful at the time, it taught me to ask these patients for an emergency contact number to add to their patient profile in case things went sideways.

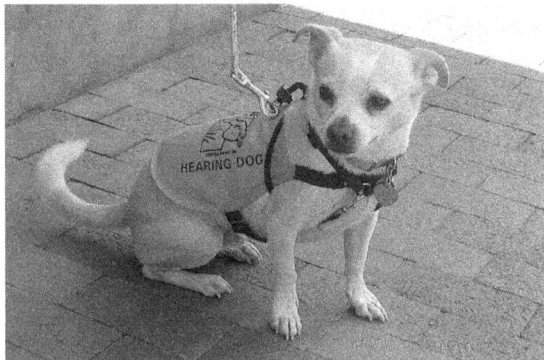

SERVICE ANIMAL POLICY

Of course, we all love a service dog. What's not to like? They're smart, well behaved, and are helping a human in need. Granted, things got a bit out of hand there for a minute with some emotional support animals. A peacock, really? I am glad these people have found something to help with their trials, but having them in a public space can sometimes be problematic.

The shops I have worked at all had some sort of policy regarding these furry companions. We would keep a bowl of fresh water outside for them on hot days, and even hemp treats behind the counter for when they visited with their humans. But unfortunately, sometimes the situation calls for what is in the best interest for patients as a whole, and not just the individual.

———

Once we had a woman come in with a purse pooch under her arm without any certification or service animal documents that would accommodate our policy. Yet nonetheless she was allowed entry by reception and proceeded to plop that puppy right on the glass top of one of our display cases.

So, I kindly asked her to either keep the dog in her arms or on the floor. You would think that I was threatening to take the mutt if she did not comply with the way she reacted. "Don't you DARE touch her!" she yelled while snatching the animal off the glass. "She has every right to be here! Just like I do!" the woman boasted. Trying to calm both the situation and my expression, I explained that in fact the dog had zero privileges due to the lack of paperwork, and that she never should have made it into the room because of this. And before she could spew more of her fantasy rights, I told her that having the dog on the actual counter was what I had an issue with. "Why? She isn't hurting anything!" the woman whined. I was losing my patience with this woman that couldn't see any farther than the tip of her own surgically sculpted nose.

"Because some people can have allergies to dogs, ma'am. And not only that, but medicine is also dispensed over this counter. It's not very sanitary to have a dog on the counter. You are not our only patient, and we pride ourselves on a safe and clean environment for everyone that visits."

With a snarky "my dog is not dirty," she was passed off to a budtender for a consultation. She was also reminded again on her way out that next time the dog would not be allowed into the med room without proper documentation. I headed for the receptionist to deliver a speech about how the situation never should have happened, and why we had the policies that we did.

SECURITY

Anyone who has ever walked into a pot shop can clearly see that every square inch of the place is being monitored by cameras. As it should be. These locations have a deeper concern for the possibility of being knocked over than, say, a liquor store. If a party store is robbed it's usually for the cash, lottery tickets, and smokes. The thieves are not looking to snag booze-based inventory because there generally isn't a resale demand. You are not likely to find the sale of individual shots of vodka on the street corners any time soon (I'd hope). But with cannabis, the bandit can easily break it down and distribute it.

Having had marijuana illegal for so long, we have all been conditioned to the idea that law enforcement are the bad guys. And in turn, I believe they have always seen us as the bad guys. Both sides have to stop thinking this way within the regulated market. Every single place that I have worked at understood that we needed to be at the very least friendly with our local law enforcement. I won't lie. It is uncomfortable at first for both sides, but neither are going anywhere, so we might as well support each other.

I encourage retail owners to invite them in! Be proud and show off your state-of-the-art beast of a safe! Brag about your key fob entry security system that you paid out your eyes for! Show them exactly what is going on and diffuse any preconceived notions of wrongdoing.

I once gave a local sheriff a tour, and I made sure to point out the age demographic in the room. They weren't degenerates or kingpins. They were middle-aged professionals looking for a bit of grease for the tin man's joints and grandparents hoping to purchase a couple of z's for the night. I also suggest that you set up some sort of an informational meet and greet with the local po-po. They can tell your staff what to expect and how to react if in fact the place is robbed or if there is a dangerous situation. Your staff in turn can let the police in on their concerns and questions when it comes to cannabis access within the shared community.

—

Now on the subject of employee safety, a set-in-stone policy has to be implemented. Especially in the case of delivery drivers and split shifts, your employees could be coming and going throughout the day. Requiring employees to use the buddy system is the best policy, in my opinion. Yep, it can be a pain in the ass waiting for someone to walk you out, but there is safety in numbers just in case someone is casing the joint.

COMMON MEDICAL CONDITIONS AND ATTRIBUTES

There are a few standard medical conditions that will cross a cannabis retail threshold on a daily basis. But what often is not considered are the behaviors that go hand-in-hand with the condition.

—

Getting to the root of the problem with patients can be quite a challenge. While some people cannot shut up about their medical issues, with others it is like pulling teeth. It is this latter type of patient who you must gently obtain certain information from if you are going to try to help them to the best of your ability. Knowing how to address not only the ailment, but the behaviors associated with them, will only make your job easier and more productive for both you and the patient.

Chronic Pain

This is such a broad category that when someone responds that they are standing at your counter due to chronic pain, it really doesn't tell you anything at all. Is it from playing football in their high school glory days, or is it from recently diagnosed MS? Both of these examples come with their own behaviors. While the former jock is cranky from day in and day out pain for decades, the MS patient is frantic with fear from their new affliction in addition to the pain.

Chronic Pain

- Chronic pain patients may walk with a cane or a limp or unbeknownst to them, physically favoring a certain part of their body.
- Paying attention to body language has a lot to do with your approach and recommendations. If you see them struggling to get across the room, offer them a chair at the counter.
- This will help to shift their attention from the pain to the conversation at hand.
- These patients can also be hard to please due to the fact they have tried every treatment under the sun, and nothing has worked.
- They find it hard to believe that cannabis will be any different. And even though their words may be cynical, the action that they took to be standing in front of you for help tells a different story.
- Some can be extremely cranky, hard to please and can have an air of superiority about them.
  - The superiority, I believe comes from the daily battle against the pain and if they are standing in front of you, they have won the day. This is great, but they are alone in this accomplishment and therefore can seem a bit haughty.
  - This is what it means to be pain-gry. Take the cranky with a grain of salt because you'd be crabby too if you were in constant pain.
  - Think about the last time you were under the weather waiting in line at the drug store for medicine that would make you feel better. You probably weren't the most personable person at the time.
  - There also must be extra consideration if the patient is trying to kick painkillers, as withdrawal symptoms are definitely a factor.
- When attempting to help those with chronic pain, asking the right questions is crucial. But it needs to be done in such a way that you are neither offensive or pushy if you wish to have any success in helping them.
- Is their pain physical (muscle or nerve issues) or is it mental/emotional (stress or anxiety related) that is the root cause of the physical pain?

- Let's say stress is keeping a patient up all night. They just can't seem to shut their head off long enough to fall asleep.
- This lack of rest causes tension headaches and achy muscles the next day from tossing and turning throughout the previous night.
- Even though a solid hybrid of cannabinoids and terpenes may help with the tensions of the day, a product heavy with myrcene or linalool can be useful for the evenings in trying to stop the awful cycle of not sleeping.
  - ☐ Once the lack of proper rest is rectified, the daily hybrid will not be necessary.
  - ☐ Always think in terms of preventative medicine. Cannabis is about taking less medication, not just more of a different kind of medicine.

Anxiety

Back in my day we called them panic attacks. In doing research for a patient, I was almost offended to find that anxiety is considered an "emotion." The panic attacks I have known felt nothing short of 100% physical. I could hear my own heartbeat in my ears, I broke out in a cold sweat, and I always felt woozy on my own feet. Anyone who has experienced panic or anxiety attacks knows that they are all encompassing, regardless of if their triggers are known.

Then there are those that are saddled with daily and uncontrollable anxiety, and the more you employ the following methods to your interactions, the better off the patient will be.

Anxeity

- Anxiety patients may speak extremely fast, ask continuous questions, or avoid eye contact to remove the attention from themselves as quickly as possible.
  - ☐ Once you determine the needs of the patient, I have found it soothing to the patient if you just ramble on about a topic while you are putting their order together.
  - ☐ This is a great opportunity to educate the patient while taking the focus off of them.
- Rapid-fire questioning may seem like accusatory behavior, but in fact is how some people handle their social situations.
- If the patient returns consistently, you'll find less and less of these behaviors as they begin to feel "safe" in your environment.
- When recommending cannabis to anxiety patients, it is very much a delicate balance. While some terpenes can double up on the paranoia, others mellow them out.

- Strong journaling by the individual and solid patient notes in your POS should cut down on the discovery period.
- Pay extra attention to which terpenes have been sampled by the patient, as some can actually make anxiety way worse.
- New-to-Cannabis patients should always start with CBD and slowly add THC. This is assuming the patient isn't taking any drugs that will negatively interact.
- When anxiety patients have an "even" day (no waves of anxiety) they feel better about their condition and worry less in the evening, making it easier to fall asleep at night.
  - ☐ A consultant should focus on finding the right product to reduce the daytime "waves".
  - ☐ Once accomplished, there will be less of a need for the nighttime products.
- It is common for those with anxiety to suffer stomach issues due to the constant stress and worry.
  - ☐ If available, CBG is showing promise for dealing with stomach issues and can be introduced with the same level of confidence as CBD, as it is also a nonintoxicating cannabinoid.

Opioid Addiction

Consulting a recovering addict can be a challenge, as there is no way of knowing where that person is in their recovery. It could have been less than 24 hours since their last fix, or they could be storing a 10-years-clean coin in their front left pocket. But regardless of their current milestone, they all must be treated with concern and respect, even if they are not returning the favor.

Opioid Addiction

- Addicts may lose focus or interest in the present moment.
  - ☐ You may find that you must repeat yourself over and over and over again.
- There may be several mood swings or behavioral changes and the patient may become pushy or unfriendly for no reason.
  - ☐ Try to adapt as seamlessly as possible and do not take it personally.
  - ☐ Their "switch" may flick back and forth several times throughout the consultation.
  - ☐ Of course, if the patient is totally out of line, you have to shut it down. You shouldn't be bullied just for trying to help someone who is struggling.

- Distorted perception of reality can happen just as quickly as the mood swings.
    - ☐ Information that was accepted at the beginning of the conversation can turn into a lie or a scam, in their mind.
        - ὑ Ex: The $15 price tag on that pre-roll was a reasonable price to them until they are asked to pay for the product. "You said it was..." is not uncommon with these consults.

Depression

We have all felt a little down in the dumps from time to time. But for some depression is a constant, crushing weight.

Consultants may have trouble with recommendations for these patients when "everything hurts." As general as this statement may be, there are answers in there, you just need to ask the right questions.

Depression

- Some patients suffer depression by sleeping for days on end, while others spend days at a time staring at the idiot box.
    - ☐ Ask the patient if the symptoms of their depression seem more prevalent during the day or at night. This distinction will help guide you in your recommendations.
        - ὑ The constant slumbering patient may benefit from products with low levels of pinene or limoneme (uplifting) and CBD for its mood-altering potential.
        - ὑ This recommendation may help the patient to stave off naps during the day and therefore may help them to achieve a healthier sleep pattern.
        - ὑ But don't forget to remind them not to take these products too late in the day, as they may cause problems with falling asleep.
    - ☐ The unmotivated, boob tube watching patient may benefit from products that have higher amount of the above mentioned pinene and limonene.
    - ☐ These may get and keep this patient alert and moving around, which may promote feelings of accomplishment.
        - ὑ Statements such as "I know, I know" and "I doubt it will do any good" are very common during these discussions.
        - ὑ They are not being intentionally rude (most of the time), so it is better to gloss over these mini digs and jabs.
        - ὑ You may have to speed up your process by sharing a personal experience with the product to reassure them.

    ʊ These patients may speak or move slowly, as if they are struggling with a great physical weight and have little regard for the conversation.

- Patience is absolutely required—especially if you are busy—with these patients as any effort to rush them will only make them move slower.

- Please remember that these patients sometimes don't get much social interaction. In fact, this may be the only trip out of the house that day. Be kind.

Alzheimer's

Age-related conditions must be catered to, as this will be the majority of your patient demographic. But just because someone is of a certain age doesn't necessarily mean that they suffer from Alzheimer's. There are few common tell-tales to help you to confirm the affliction and then you can adjust your approach in a compassionate manner.

Alzheimer's

- Alzheimer's patients can struggle with the simplest of common tasks as the disease progresses. Patients may struggle with or recount their money several times. Or it may take them several tries to open a door or answer when their name is called.
  - ☐ Don't try to help with this (unless they really can't get it.)
  - ☐ They find it depressing, helpless and it just irritates them in general.
  - ☐ Just be patient with them and offer a hand when warranted.

- These patients may be hesitant to pick up jars or magazines from counters on their own. If there is something you want the to check out, hand it to them.

- They may get turned around in small spaces (losing the entrance/exit points) or simply wander away from your station and your conversation to roam around the room.
  - ☐ In this case, come out from behind the counter and roam with them. Keep the conversation and the educating going. Adapt to the patient!

- It's so easy to judge a person based on their appearance, especially if their grooming habits, clothing choices and hygiene are less than desirable.
  - ☐ Just don't.
  - ☐ Maybe this person has lost the ability to hold a toothbrush or a comb and haven't been able to admit it to themselves yet.
  - ☐ We all have a battle going on!

Patient Notes

I cannot stress the importance of solid patient notes in your POS enough. I encourage you to put in anything that you deem helpful. Maybe it's the name of a daughter that always comes in with Dad, or which branch of service the veteran was in, or how they are famous for trying to return half smoked joints (it's happened more than once).

So, even if it is only a few words, it really can help with giving everyone a heads up on a patient's preferences, behaviors, and any potential compliance or product concerns, while making the patient feel taken care of.

PRODUCT COMPLAINTS

A product doesn't have to be on your shelf for very long for you to find out if a product is problematic. When presented with a complaint, regardless of your return policy, be apologetic and offer a remedy. Consultants also need to document any complaints for the following reasons.

CHRONIC COMPLAINERS

- Some people you just can't please. Notes in the patient's file will give a consultant a heads up on how it was handled in the past. You can use the same past remedy in hopes that if this person gets the same response every time, they may stop trying the same scam.

FAULTY PRODUCTS

- It will be easier to take this issue up with the vendor if you have clear documentation showing a consistent problem with the product.

If a patient has complained about a product in the past and is attempting to buy it again, remind them that they didn't care for it the last time they bought it. People forget. Knowing at a glance what the patient has ordered in the past can help with future recommendations.

EXAMPLE

- Dan states that he has been unhappy with his last couple of flower purchases. His patient notes indicate that he has bought heavy sativas both times and is about to buy another one.
- By paying attention in this manner a budtender can recommend something more along the lines of a hybrid in hopes that Dan will be satisfied with his next purchase.

NOTES

Notes on any potential compliance issues help document and decipher if there really is something fishy going on.

- Dolly wants her quarter ounce packaged in individual grams. To me this screams "resale." I would just tell her that it is against shop policy to break up a quarter ounce into separate packages due to the possibility of resale.

- If Dolly is elderly and needs help with measuring out her dosages, you can always show her what one gram will look like and she can split it up herself.

These notes are another means of communication between budtenders that have helped the same patient.

- Jack takes his time and wanders around the room. According to his notes following him around the room will speed up his tire-kicking time.

- Jane complains at every visit about the prices and always tries to get freebies. A gentle reminder of which days have which specials quiets her demands.

REMEDIES FOR HARASSMENT AND DIFFICULT CUSTOMERS

It requires very thick skin to work in cannabis retail. I had a managing partner once ask what I mean by that. I told him that some people find that they simply do not have the stomach for it. It's a different beast of retail. Dealing with people's medical conditions and complaints can be extremely challenging day in and day out.

I have been called so many names over the years while standing behind the cannabis counter that I've lost count. But two really stick out and still make me chuckle to this day. The first one is when a woman called me a "bad apple" (hehe), because I wouldn't let her return a half-eaten edible. My other favorite is when a voluptuous family of five all wanted to come into the med room together. We had very limited space and our policy called for no more than two at a time. I told them I would make an exception and they could go back in two groups (one of two and the other of three). Unsatisfied with my efforts, I was called a "snarky bitch." I actually laughed at this guy and said, "Now I am retracting my compromise to our store policy. We only allow two back at a time." And I walked away.

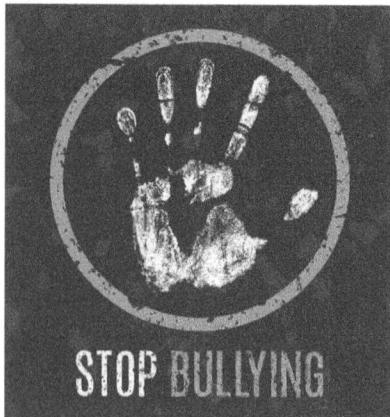

STOP BULLYING

Bullies

Bullying is a big problem in the cannabis industry. It's disgraceful that bullying has become so commonplace in cannabis that it is tolerated, and sometimes even accommodated. The same sensible edict that is granted to pharmacies, gas stations, and grocery stores, is simply not being enforced in cannabis retail.

Some cheeky patients are delusional, thinking that because they spend a certain number of dollars at your store, know somebody in the business, or because they bring a friend with them that they deserve recognition in the form of a kickback.

I don't know about you, but I drop some serious coin at the grocery store and at the gas stations every week. Yet, if I was to approach the gas station attendant, and demand that I deserve a free tank of gas because of the money I spend there, I would be laughed out of the place. And what do you think would happen if I walked up to the cashier at the grocery store and announced that I had brought my friend along, and followed it up with, "What do I get for doing that?" And heaven knows that I certainly didn't get extra pills in my prescriptions because I knew the pharmacist by name.

So, where did this notion that dispensaries work on the level as backroad flea markets come from?

Does it stem from past interactions with the black market? I highly doubt it. The fact is you didn't dicker about the price of the product with your supplier in the parking lot of the local pizza joint.

Is there a sense of entitlement by association? Bullies are famous for name-dropping, in the hopes that the budtender is either impressed or cowed by the possibility that they are "friends" with the owner or vendors in the local industry. Try again. Everyone knows "a guy." If they are so in tune with the pulse of the cannabis industry, they wouldn't be standing at a dispensary counter, giving the budtender a hard time, asking for free product.

Could it possibly be an age thing? The majority of cannabis retail employees are in their 20s, while the middle of the road for cannabis patients is their late 40s. So, do these harassing patients feel they are superior to the younger generation behind the counter? Does their advanced age warrant them that free pre-roll, and no young punk is going to deny them these self-proclaimed rights? Or is it simply because they have endured the struggle of buying their medication underground for so long? Please, not that old chestnut.

When denied, the classic five-year-old playground bully reaction will lead them to spending the rest of their consultation passively throwing little digs about the lack of quality product being offered. This is mixed in with attempts to belittle the budtender with their "expertise" in all thing's cannabis (which is usually just more bullshit and bravado). I have even observed them huffing and grumbling and shuffling their feet in a restrained form of a temper tantrum while browsing the displays. Yes, these are fully grown men and women acting this way.

Bullies can smell fear. Aggressors will take any opening to browbeat a timid employee with loud declarations of how much money they spend weekly, that they even bring friends with them to make your store more money, and how XYZ store accommodates their demands. This intimidates and wears down an unprepared budtender. It muddles their perspective of who is really calling the shots.

As this forced professional fatigue shows signs of taking its toll, this predator instinctively knows that their odds are inching them toward getting what they want. Now they lay the beratement on even thicker, pushing the counter person to turn to management to ask if they can throw in something extra. If management concedes, even if they only do so to get this unruly patient to leave the store, the bully has won. This combative victory will be twisted into "the budtender did it for me last time" in the future, and then they will proceed to run with it until the wheels fall off.

Bullies have always been a part of the retail consumer demographic and are not likely to fade away anytime soon. Therefore, proper budtender training on how to diffuse these bullies and retain a strict store policy is essential. You have to stop feeding these monsters. This is your house, own it.

So, regardless of their justifications, how is a budtender to professionally defend themselves against this increasingly popular type of harassment? The most common reaction, and the right one, is the "shut down." The following calm, canned responses will give you an idea on how to shut them down, and how you can tweak your own premeditated responses.

HARASSMENT EXAMPLES

Patient:

"I spend a lot of money in here."

Response:

We really appreciate that! That's why we have different daily discounts to reward our loyal customers.

Patient:

"I tell people to come in here all the time."

Response:

Thanks so much for that! If you happen to be with a new to us patient, we can throw a few loyalty points your way.

Patient:

"I can get it cheaper at ABC dispensary."

Response:

We all have different discounts for our customers. (Don't discredit the competition. It's petty.)

Between your referral programs, senior, veteran, and daily promotions, there is something for everyone.

If a problematic customer still cannot be calmed or deterred by some variation of the above remedies, it's up to management (when given authority) to properly shut it down. Some of the locations I have worked for used the three-strike approach, some wanted the decision to go through the higher ups, and others just left these decisions to the floor manager. I have always tried to give these types of people multiple opportunities to keep themselves off of the banned list. I've made notes in patient files to ensure that maybe a specific budtender should not be assisting a specific customer. I have stuck my nose in conversations that smell of conflict to try to neutralize the situation, and I have even asked, "you like coming here, don't you? You would like to continue to, wouldn't you?" If these didn't work and the customer was still aggressive, I would make sure that they understood what the consequences would be.

—

I was plugging away at my managerial mountain of emails in my office when Penny knocked on my door to tell me that she was fed up with the customer she was trying to help. She explained that the guy kept taking age-related jabs at her, and was combative to the point of taking products out of his basket and tossing them back behind the counter like he was sifting through a recycling bin. She finally told him that she had to run in the back to do a price check just to regain her patience and let me know what was up. Penny was a solid employee that could always handle whatever situation arose. So, the fact that she was in my doorway and at a loss with this guy spoke volumes.

Setting my correspondence aside, I followed her back out onto the floor to assess the situation for myself by straightening a shelf within earshot. She had barely bellied back up to her station when the guy said, "Needed someone to do the math for you, didn't you? I'm not surprised. None of you kids know how to count without your fingers."

Penny cooly responded with, "Not at all. I was checking to see if yesterday's flower discount still applied. It doesn't." This guy took this as free passage to continue to berate my budtender.

"Why would you try to sell me any then? You're a special kind of stupid, aren't you?"

That was all I needed to hear.

I walked up next to Penny, took this guy's basket filled with his selections, and put it under the counter. "You're done. We are not here for you to beat up just because you are having a bad day and need someone to take it out on. We are only here to help. I will not have anyone treating my employees the way I heard you just treating Penny here." With eyes as wide as saucers, he began to sputter and whine that she wasn't doing this, and she wasn't doing that. Grabbing his name with a glance at the screen, I continued with, "Mr. Otto you are no longer welcome here. You are banned. There's the door. Use it." Like an overgrown spoiled brat in the grocery store, he began to yell "This place sucks! Everything here is trash! You all are just so ... so ... useless!" as he stormed out the door. I told Penny to put detailed notes in his profile about the interaction and add "banned" in red capital letters at the top with my initials for authorization.

———

Some days later, Penny gave me the nod toward the lobby as Mr. Otto was trying to check in. This ought to be good, I thought as I headed for the door. I directed the guy into the corner of the lobby just in case he wanted to cause a scene again. "What part of 'banned' didn't you understand? Are you going to start ranting and raving again at our customers Mr. Otto? Because if you are, I have no problem calling the police," I said, crossing my arms over my chest. Mr. Otto put his hands up in a defensive position as he explained that he was in fact having a bad day the last time. And that he was so very sorry, and if I could give him another chance, he'd never do it again. I wasn't completely convinced that this guy even realized what he had done wrong to earn himself the banishment in the first place.

So, I thought to get creative. "I tell you what. The budtender that you used as a verbal punching bag the last time just happens to be working today. I will leave this decision up to her. I'll let her know that you would like to speak with her. She may come out, she may not. You can plead your case with her and if she is in a forgiving mood, I will lift the ban. If she isn't, and I wouldn't blame her, the ban stays."

So that is exactly what I did. I gave Penny the lowdown on how I wanted to handle this situation and that I was good with whatever she decided. I also recommended that she made the guy sweat it out for at least 20 minutes if she did decide to hear him out. No point in giving priority to people like that, I thought as

I returned to my desk. I never saw how much time Penny spent in the lobby, but I did check Mr. Otto's profile at the end of the day which read "ban lifted" in green with the date and my initials.

Boss Bullies

Bully status isn't just reserved for customers. There is a large bullying problem with the owners of some of these cannabis companies as well. You will find crazy turnover numbers in the cannabis space, because when you treat someone like they are disposable, this is exactly how they will act. Some of the bosses I have known over the years have been scam artists, dirtbags, cowards, and narcissists of biblical proportions.

———

Working for owners that have never run a staff or have never had employees of their own is quite problematic. They have no clue on how to juggle single moms, young adults in college, or those that are caretakers for disabled or aging relatives. They do not see their employees as human, but as property. In fact, the majority of issues that I have had in the cannabis-retail space stem from the higher ups treating their employees like cattle.

These examples of crappy human behavior have ranged from owners threatening termination if employees were found to be socializing after hours, to being banned from having any contact at all with someone that was a former employee. As if they owned these people's lives completely.

I have witnessed a newly pregnant mother go from 30 hours a week to 5 hours once the owners were notified of her condition. They have scheduled single moms with little ones to work on Halloween night and Christmas Eve (even when they weren't normal scheduled days), while giving their family members two weeks off for the holiday. Paid. I have applauded CEOs for hiring the handicapped only to find that months later they had forced this person to complete a task that they were clearly physically incapable of carrying out. When I pushed back, their response was, "if they can't do it, they can't work here."

People have quietly resigned just to have the owners hold their last paycheck until the former employees had to retain an attorney to get what was owed.

I have witnessed an owner just hours away from shutting down the business without so much as a heads up to their employees (mostly single parents and college kids). The response was, "they'll find out when they show up for work tomorrow."

I have stated very clearly to every single cannabis company I have worked for, subcontracted or not, that I will remain loyal and work tirelessly (in some cases pulling close to 80 hours a week) as long as they are not hurting anyone. Simple enough, right?

But unfortunately, more times than not, once these owners began to make a couple of bucks, they lost sight of the mantra that had me wanting to work for them in the first place. "Patients over Profits" t-shirts were worn while the staff was forced to remove expiration dates from products, and parading a physically disabled child in advertisements to bring traffic in the door. As the old saying goes, a financial windfall will make good people better and bad people worse. So, for those of you that like to pass judgment on employment turnover or those that think they have me pegged because I have worked for several different cannabis companies over the years, know that the above examples are only the "reader friendly" ones. I still stand by my reasons for moving on. I absolutely refuse to work for garbage human beings.

FIRST CONSULT WITH NEW-TO-CANNABIS CONSUMERS

Employees must recognize that they have a responsibility to the consumer to offer educated information. If you find yourself unsure, it is always better to say that you don't know than give false information. Employees should also never, ever use the "C" word. No, not that one, but the word "cure." There simply isn't enough research to support this claim, and the last thing you want to do is give someone false hope. But what we can say is that cannabis has the potential to help with the right conditions. When speaking about what cannabis may do for someone, I have always found it best to stick with the following phrases.

RECOMMENDATIONS AND RESPONSIBILITY
Employees should use phrases such as:

"I have personally found ..."

"Current research suggests ..."

"Patients have reported ..."

Cite credible references.

The first few questions you ask new-to-cannabis consumers are critical if you are going to help this person to the best of your ability.

NEW TO CANNABIS PATIENTS

- Have you tried cannabis before?
- How did you take it?
- What are you looking to use cannabis for?
- Do you have any allergies or are you diabetic?
- What effects do you *not* want?
- Have you spoken with your doctors about cannabis?
- Do you take any drugs that have a grapefruit warning?

I learned the weight-of-my-words lesson the hard way. I was speaking to a group at a local American House on the very basics of using cannabis as medicine. This included a bit on how CBD can be compared to an anti-inflammatory like Advil or Motrin, but should not be purchased from gas stations, but state-licensed facilities after getting permission from their doctors. After my presentation

I packed up and made my way back to the shop. Before I had even made it a mile down the road, I had the director of the facility calling me to say there was an irate family member wanting to speak with me. I racked my brain on the way back to the facility about what I could've possibly have said to get a family member all wound up!

—

It turned out that the very, very angry gentleman's mother was in attendance for my presentation and took my information about CBD to mean quite literally that she could stop taking all of her pills if she could just get a ride to the gas station. Dementia is a jerk. No wonder this guy was livid. Both the director and I gushed apologies and explained what was actually said, and that it was his mother that had gotten it twisted around. Of course, this didn't matter to the son as we could all hear his mother continuing to holler from the second floor about a ride to the gas station.

It just goes to show that you can say and do all of the right things and stupid shit can still happen.

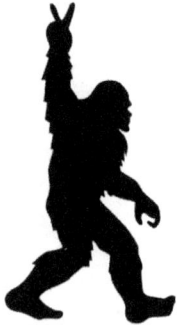

Legends, half-truths, and nonsense

With the constant swirl of pot politics and celebrity endorsements, some truly amazing pioneers are not getting the limelight I believe they deserve. I will try to do them some justice in the following section, which also includes how misinformation in the cannabis industry isn't only reserved for the effects that it can have on the human condition. There are a ton of urban legends that have been created by the storyteller stoners over the decades. Some have merit, some were based on a truth at some point, and others are just complete hogwash.

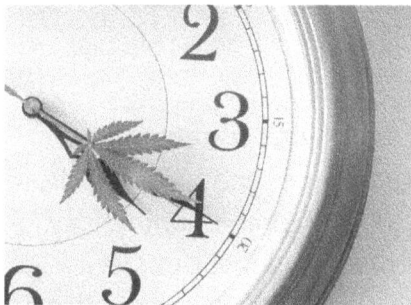

420

Oh, the wonder of our beloved holiday! Live music, food trucks, bundle deals, and freebies as far as our red eyes can see. Retailers spend months planning for the 20th day of April—and for good reason. 420 is often explained as the St. Paddy's Day for stoners (minus the car bomb shots and vomit), and brings in crowds from far and wide. The last time I worked retail on a 420, it was a slushy, nasty Michigan day, yet we still saw over 500 people. Many a midnight toker has spent their day bouncing around to the different dispensaries to collect as much free stuff as they possibly can. These goodies can range from bud to Bic lighters and bandanas—with purchase of course.

In preparation for the circus ahead of us, I had asked my staff that morning to retell the story of how the holiday got its roots, as the question would be asked over and over again throughout the day. I have to say that I was a bit disappointed to find that not one of the dozen stoners in front of me really knew, so I gathered them around for the details behind the folklore.

It is easy to get this story wrong, as there are many variations and urban legends surrounding the date and its meaning. Some believe that it is the number of active chemicals in Marijuana (NIH states 540)[134], some reference it to Hitler's birthday (in 1889), and others credit Bob Dylan and his tune "Rainy Day Woman No. 12 & 35" for the lyrics "everybody must get stoned," because 12 multiplied by 35 does, in fact equal 420.[135] And if you are a baseball fan, you should know that both Fenway and Tiger Stadium both opened on April 20th, 1912.[136]

—

But the reality is that the roots of the 420 legend can be traced back to five teenage athletes who attended San Rafael High School in California. In true stoner simplicity, they coined themselves "The Waldos" from the way they would hang out on campus. They had caught wind in the fall of 1971 that a member of the Coast Guard had planted a crop of unattended weed in the area, and it was even said that there was a "treasure" map drawn by the coastie himself. So, the quintet began meeting at the Louis Pasteur statue outside of the school at 4:20 p.m. at least once a week in search of the field of green. They never did find the unsecured crop, but the term 420 stuck around, as a way for teens to reference pot without the adults being any the wiser.[137]

---

[134]https://www.nccih.nih.gov/health/cannabis-marijuana-and-cannabinoids-what-you-need-to-know
[135]https://www.history.com/news/the-hazy-history-of-420
[136]https://sports.yahoo.com/news/tiger-stadium-opened-100-years-ago-just-like-fenway-park--but-it-s-ignored-in-detroit.html
[137]https://www.history.com/news/the-hazy-history-of-420

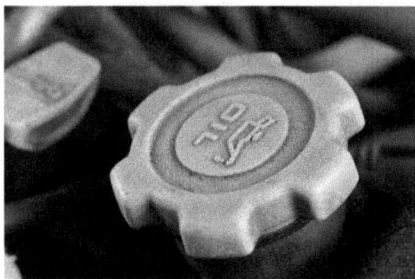

710

July 10th (7/10) is a fairly new holiday in the stoner culture. It comes with most of the fanfare that 420 does, but it does cater to a younger crowd. It is a day to celebrate and partake in concentrates, a.k.a oil. If you take the word "OIL" and turn it upside down, you get "710." That's it. That's the whole story. It's not rocket science folks, and I feel like there should be a blonde joke in there somewhere.

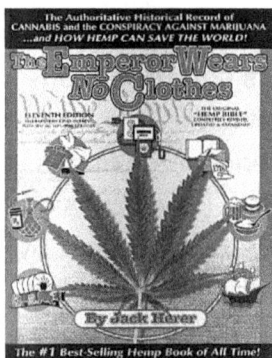

Jack Herer (June 18, 1939 – April 15, 2010)

When one speaks of true cannabis activism and the fight for legalization, Jack Herer should be on the top of the list. He has been called the "Emperor of Hemp" and the "Godfather of the cannabis movement" and even has a very popular cannabis strain named after him. In 1985 he wrote the now classic *The Emperor Wears No Clothes*, which has been used to motivate and inspire those looking to continue to fight for hemp derived medicine, food, and fiber.[138]

What Jack had started is still celebrated with the competition of The Jack Herer Cup held each year in Columbia, Amsterdam, Las Vegas, and Oklahoma City.[139]

My favorite quote from the man is, "Hemp will be the future of all mankind, or there won't be a future." I don't think he's wrong.

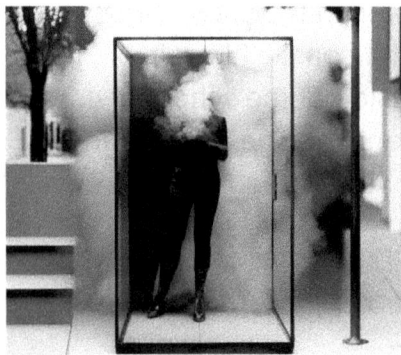

Hotboxing

If you have ever seen the cult classic *Fast Times at Ridgemont High*, you will remember the scene where all the guys pile out of the van in a cloud of smoke. This is known as hotboxing. It is the act of confining yourself in a space that exposes you to a heavy amount of secondhand cannabis smoke. There are many that are afraid of getting a "contact high," or popping positive on a drug test just

---

[138]https://www.jackherer.com/
[139]https://en.wikipedia.org/wiki/Jack_Herer#cite_note-2

from being around this smoke. So, can someone catch a buzz just by being in the same room as someone smoking a joint?

"Researchers measured the amount of THC in the blood of people who do not smoke marijuana and had spent 3 hours in a well-ventilated space with people casually smoking marijuana; THC was present in the blood of the non-smoking participants, but the amount was well below the level needed to fail a drug test. Another study that varied the levels of ventilation and the potency of the marijuana found that some non-smoking participants exposed for an hour to high-THC marijuana (11.3% THC concentration) in an unventilated room showed positive urine assays in the hours directly following exposure; a follow-up study showed that nonsmoking people in a confined space with people smoking high-THC marijuana reported mild subjective effects of the drug—a 'contact high'—and displayed mild impairments on performance in motor tasks."[140]

If you are concerned with having THC in your system, small amounts or not, I suggest that you remove yourself from the space. Better safe than sorry.

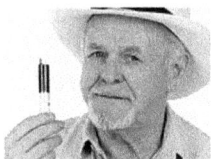

Rick Simpson

Just about everyone into cannabis for medical reasons has heard of RSO (aka Rick Simpson Oil). If you haven't, it's a highly concentrated, dark, sticky, diabolical-looking product usually packaged in syringes or capsules.

Rick Simpson was an engineer from Canada who had suffered a head injury in 1997, and due to the side effects of his prescribed pills, he went looking for an alternative solution. He began using extractions from the cannabis he grew in his own backyard, and it seemed to do the trick. So, he took it upon himself to share his story, give away the concoction (and recipe) for free, and became an activist for legal access to medical marijuana.[141]

In 2003 Rick was diagnosed with a common skin cancer and thought to use the same tar-like substance topically to see if it would help. He claims that it cleared up his cancer in just four days, and though recent research does not necessarily support the short time frame, it is showing promise as a treatment for skin cancer.

---

[140]NIDA. 2021, April 13. What are the effects of secondhand exposure to marijuana smoke?. Retrieved from https://nida.nih.gov/publications/research-reports/marijuana/what-are-effects-secondhand-exposure-to-marijuana-smoke on 2023, March 16
[141]https://www.wikileaf.com/thestash/rick-simpson-oil/

Because people can be just the absolute worst, there are plenty of fake RSO sites out there riding on the coattails of Mr. Simpson. According to his original site, Phoenix Tears, he is only affiliated with www.simpsonramadur.com and www.phoenixtears.ca

Henry Ford's Hemp Car

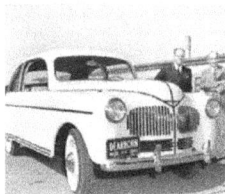

Funny how a girl that was born and raised in the Motor City, where just about everyone's employment was tied to the automotive industry in some fashion, had to extend her reach all the way south of the Mason Dixon Line to get the truth about a car.

Now, I have seen plenty of publications and documentaries on Henry Ford's famous "hemp car" over the years, but when gathering information on the subject I had found that none of them seemed to match. So, I reached out to the distinguished author of *Tales from the Kentucky Hemp Highway*, Dan Isenstein, for some clarification from a true hemp historian.

Dan has been gracious enough to contribute the following summary on the subject, and if the history of hemp's use in the US sparks your interest, be sure to check out his book!

Henry Ford's Hemp Car That Wasn't

There is a popular legend that in the 1930s Henry Ford grew hemp so he could make a car out of hemp that ran on hemp fuel. Thanks to the internet, this is a widely circulated story, but how much of this legend is true and how much is just hempsters blowing smoke?

Interest in exploring non-food uses for crops started to gain favor in the years following the First World War, and reached its peak during the Great Depression, especially in the years just preceding the United States' entry into the Second World War. The advocates of this new avenue of scientific investigation believed that through chemistry, America's agricultural bounty could be converted into the raw materials for countless products from fuel to plastics.

The promise of converting agricultural produce into alternative fuels and raw materials for manufacturing caught the attention of Henry Ford. Ford's interest in the potential of chemistry and the farm to supply the materials required to manufacture and power automobiles helped to provide scientists with a great deal of credibility. This interest culminated in the production of a prototype vehicle, and legend has it this car was made from and powered by hemp.

While many toiled developing "nonfood uses for crops," the new field of science was not named "chemurgy" until 1934 when William J. Hale, an important figurehead of the Dow Chemical Corporation, wrote the highly influential book *The Farm Chemurgic*.

Ford saw potential in the chemurgic movement and on May 7, 1935, the first National Chemurgic conference was held at his research lab in Dearborn.

The conference identified developing a fuel-alcohol product, "Agrol," as the top priority for the council. Initially conceived and proposed as a gasoline additive, "Agrol" was developed to eliminate knocks and increase octane. However, the leadership of the National Farm Chemurgic, namely Garvan and Hale, were outspoken in their almost religious belief that fuel-alcohol could eventually replace gasoline altogether in internal combustion engines.

The obstacles facing the development of fuel-alcohol were substantial. The sometimes antagonistic and outlandish statements made by some of the council's leaders made them worse. A project of such scope required partners both in government and the private sector. But, both Francis Garvan of the Chemical Foundation and Hale had made powerful enemies; Garvan vocally targeted the petroleum industry, while Hale was an outspoken critic of the US Department of Agriculture.

While the fuel alcohol project was the council's focus, research into alternative manufacturing materials was the second priority. Ford was personally interested in finding new materials that could replace imported raw materials like rubber and expensive domestically produced materials like steel.

In 1941, just prior to World War II, Ford's in-house team completed a prototype vehicle. The car was built on a tubular steel frame and incorporated phenolic resin body panels embedded with natural fibers, which included among other things hemp, flax, and kenaf. It was designed to run on Agrol. A second prototype under construction at the outbreak of the Second World War was scrapped as Ford and the rest of the nation dedicated its manufacturing capacity to the war effort. Likewise, all chemurgic research was now devoted to supporting the war effort. The first prototype was also destroyed.

The manufacturing process used to make plastic body panels for Ford's prototype was time-consuming and would have been inefficient for large scale production. The narrative that there was significant hemp content in Ford's chemurgic car is simply not true. Hemp comprised an extremely small proportion of the prototype vehicle produced.

The premise that "anything made from plastic can be made of hemp," is essentially meme bait simply paraphrasing a concept Hale considered core to "chemurgy," that anything made from a "hydrocarbon" (petroleum) could be made from a "carbohydrate" (plant matter). Research into developing industrial raw materials from organic material or agricultural products continues to this day. No longer called "chemurgy," this field of research is now called "biomechanical engineering."

If there were truly more to the story of Henry Ford's "hemp plastic car that runs on hemp fuel," it would be more than a meme. The idea of a "hemp" car or a "hemp" airplane inspires the imagination, but the reality of hemp-based manufacturing materials is that they were and currently remain a novelty.

Uekotter, Frank. The Revolt of the Chemists: biofuels, agricultural overproduction and the chemurgy movement in New Deal America History and Technology, 37:4, pg. 431 Pursell, Carroll W. The Farm Chemurgic Council and the United States Department of Agriculture, 1935-1939 Isis, Vol. 60 No. 3 Autumn 1969 pg. 310 Ibid; 309

Uekotter, Frank. The Revolt of the Chemists: biofuels, agricultural overproduction and the chemurgy movement in New Deal America History and Technology, 37:4, pp. 435-436

Van Duyne, Schulyer. Henry Ford Demonstrates Plastic Bodies for Cars Popular Science March 1941

Harris, Kathryn. New Book on Henry Ford Libel Trial Sheds Light on History of Hate Speech https://www.americanbarfiundation.org/news/345 June 14, 2012 accessed March 8, 2023

Uekotter, Frank. The Revolt of the Chemists: biofuels, agricultural overproduction, and the chemurgy movement in New Deal America History and Technology, 37:4, 429-445, DOI

Ganzel, Bill. Postwar Economic Boom Affects Farmers Wessel's Living History Farm https://livinghistoryfarm.org/farminginthe40s/money_11.html accessed March 7, 2023

Manaia, João P., Ana T. Manaia, and Lúcia Rodriges. 2019. "Industrial Hemp Fibers: An Overview" Fibers 7, no. 12: 106. https://doi.org/10.3390/fib7120106 accessed March 22, 2023

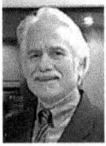

Richard Rose

I have been a fan of Richard Rose since the beginning of my career in cannabis. Initially, it wasn't for his hard-core entrepreneurship or the historical changes that he impressed upon our food industry (which I was ignorant of until now), but his humanity. His honest sincerity to help his fellow humans.

Forty years ago, Richard started an entire crusade, which became hemp's first billion-dollar industry, by being the first to bring smart-branded foods made from hemp seed to the masses. Coined the "Tofu Mogul," and rightfully so, having also been the first to offer such products as vegan eggnog (1981), tofu frozen dessert powdered mixes (1985), tofu ice cream exported to Japan (1986), organic vegan cream cheese (1994), and all while running the first vegan restaurant in California in 1980.[142] Whew!

—

As if he didn't have enough going on, Richard decided to shift his focus to hemp in 1994. Hemp was a better source of protein and had been around long enough to support this claim. So, why not replace the soy in our food industry with shelled hemp seeds? And since nobody was importing non-sterilized hemp seeds at the time, he put his million-dollar businesses and his freedom on the line to introduce shelled hempseed to North America.

This accomplishment earned him another title as "The Hemp Nut," named after his company HempNut Inc., which between 1994–2002 was groundbreaking for creating the best practices for hemp seed foods in North America. Richard's products were so on point that his "Hempeh Burger" had an FDA health claim that it actually reduced the risk of heart disease.[143] That commendation didn't just fall in his lap, he earned it.

[142]https://www.higherlearninglv.co/post/the-higher-learning-lv-interview-richard-rose
[143]https://therichardrosereport.com/1994-hempeh-burger/

In true Mr. Rose style, he continued to cross the finish line first with hemp food sold in a military PX (1996), introducing shelled hempseed to the US and Canada (1996), and organizing a 27-member international supply chain to export hempseed to Europe, Canada, Japan, China, and Australia.[144]

———

Then, as if Richard wasn't doing enough to help the health of his fellow humans, he added CBD to his revolutionary resume. He created "Nobacco" and "Not-Pot," which are made out of craft hemp flower that can be smoked. He started the Medicinal Hemp Association, the Hemp Flower Products Association, and even brought the Hemp Food Association back from the grave.

Even with decades of noble accomplishments, my favorite thing about Mr. Rose is that he is always willing to teach, always willing to share his knowledge and ideas regardless of where you are on the totem pole of life. To this end, he has created a free cannabis library (CannLib) with over twenty thousand PDFs relating to cannabis and offers "CannaSearch," which grants access to the cannabis research of 64 different medical conditions so people can learn for themselves.[145]

Of course, anyone who has been in the cannabis industry for long enough cannot help but to have a sense of humor, and Richard is no different. When asked during an interview with *Hemp Today* if they could call him a "guru," Richard responded with, "I've been called far worse by those engaged in f***ery of the first order. But if you insist, call me "CannGuru" ... I have all kinds of ideas in my pouch."[146] I'm willing to bet the hemp farm that he does.

---

[144]https://therichardrosereport.com/articles2/richard-rose-professional-history/
[145]https://therichardrosereport.com/about/
[146]https://hemptoday.net/richard-rose-interview/

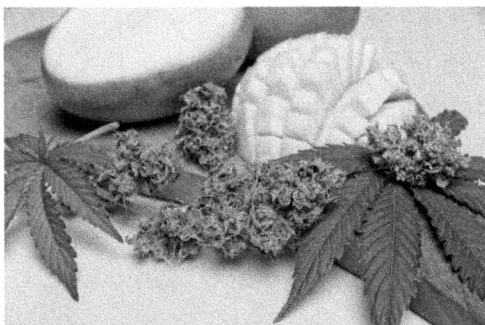

"Mangoes Increase Your High."

Most of us have heard this one. It is the theory that if you combine mangos with your cannabis intake you will get higher because you are doubling down on the terpene myrcene. Although that mango smoothie you have is extra yummy and does a fine job at squashing your cottonmouth, it isn't enhancing your buzz. Contrary to popular belief, mangos really don't contain high concentrations of myrcene, and what myrcene it does have is not housed in the fleshy fruit, but in the skin. And if you were thinking about eating just the skin of a mango, I'd listen to the following warning by Dr. Codi Peterson, "... mangoes contain urushiol, the same compound present in poison ivy and poison oak. So don't start eating mango skins to get extra high or you're likely to bite off more than you bargained for."[147]

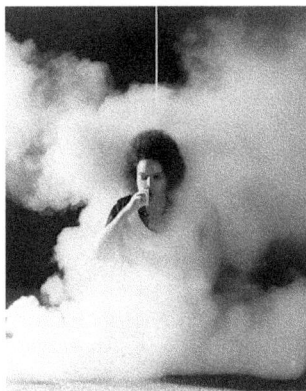

"Holding Your Hit Gets You Higher."

There is a fairytale that the longer you hold your toke the higher you will get. I'm here to tell you that all of your eye-watering, red-faced choking is for not.

How high you get from smoking cannabis has more to do with THC potency than the actual time spent holding your breath. This is because when THC is inhaled, it heads straight to the alveoli (air sacs in the lungs), and any available cannabinoids will be absorbed within mere seconds and then pushed in the direction of your bloodstream. Holding your breath past this point is only holding on to the harmful byproducts and carcinogens of smoking.[148]

Stop it.

---

[147] https://cannigma.com/physiology/foods-that-can-affect-your-high/
[148] https://cannigma.com/cannabis-news/does-holding-cannabis-smoke-in-longer-make-a-difference/

A Stoner Love Story

I couldn't say what day of the week it was, but I do remember the vibe in the room. We were all beat up from the feet up by patients and technology pushing us around all day. We had endured everything from the ATM spitting out fives instead of twenties (the keys were M.I.A.), to a woman ranting that the topical we sold her gave her diarrhea, and when asked if she actually ate the topical, she responded with smashing a tip jar on the floor before stomping out. Mama said there would be days like this.

I had just sent our receptionist for a much-needed break after another relentless rush, and the closest budtender gladly took her place simply for the opportunity to sit and rest her barking dogs. With everyone on the floor doing some sort of recouping, I took the next patient to give them some additional time.

My customer service tank was running on fumes, but I still managed a "Hi darling. What brings you in?" The tall, Dean Martin-look-alike before me answered that he was hurting from building a firepit all day and could use a few pre-rolls for the pain.

I turned towards the shelves that held the glass jars filled with our offerings when he added with a voice like a bass drum, "got anything that won't make me cough?" Speaking over my shoulder, I matched his question with one of my own.

"Are you holding in your hit?"

"Well, yeah. That's how we were taught to do it in middle school," he answered with dimples tugging at the corners of his smile.

Handsome or not, I was in no mood for playful banter and snapped back with, "Stop listening to 7th graders. The only thing you are holding in are the carcinogens from the smoke. Any of the good stuff gets into your lungs much faster than you would think. Plus holding your breath, even without smoke in your lungs, will get you lightheaded. So, if your argument is that it gets you higher, try again."

I didn't give him the opportunity to reply, and I moved the interaction along by picking out two pre-rolls that were a bit smoother than the others. As I went to ring him up, he informed me that his bank card wasn't working and sheepishly handed me a double, large-handed fistful of quarters. And why not? This was how the whole day had been. But I honestly didn't care at this point. It wasn't my money after all, as long as it added up. With a Lili Von Shtupp "I'm so tired" smile, I sent him on his way.

A few days later he came back to let me know that he did try my advice on how to properly smoke a joint and that he did indeed cough less. Requesting a few more of the same pre-rolls that he purchased earlier that week, he not only relayed that he had "folding money" this time, but would like to hangout and scribbled his number on a flyer on the counter.

Maybe it was the boyish dimpled grin, or his gravelly voice, or maybe it was because he could actually build things with his own two hands (honestly, who does that anymore), that got my attention.

———

I no longer question the fates about how I was found by my knight in shining armor in a pot shop, cranky as hell. Because regardless, to this very day I am so thankful that he was still using middle school ministry and that my brand of snark didn't deter him. He has been making me sway for years now, and after suffering through a few of my "respect the herb" speeches and getting him to ditch the homemade pop can pipes, I am still absolutely smitten with the man that is the love of my life.

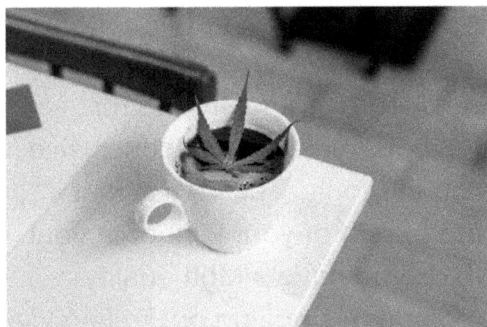

Wake and Bake

If you don't know the term, it is when you smoke cannabis first thing when you wake up. If you smoke with your morning cuppa Joe, it is called a "hippie speedball."

Partaking within the first hour of waking up is more popular than one might think. A global drug survey from 2017 shows that Americans have the highest rate of any country at 21.9%. Mexico is next in line at 18.4%, Greece is at 15.9%, our brother to the north comes in at 14.9%, and lastly Brazil at 14.3%.[149]

---

[149]https://www.globaldrugsurvey.com/wp-content/themes/globaldrugsurvey/results/GDS2017_key-find-ings-report_final.pdf

---

People report that when doing this they feel "higher," and for a longer period of time than if they were to consume later in the day. Some guess that the reason is because you are still sleepy or that your body hasn't moved around any nutrients during your slumber. But a more scientific approach to the question might be closer to the truth.

At this point you know that our ECS is a regulator. This also includes our circadian rhythm (our internal clock that tells us when we are hungry and when to fall asleep and wake up).

According to an article scientifically reviewed by Codi Peterson, PharmD, "Research has shown that the amounts of all three components of the ECS—endocannabinoids, receptors, and enzymes—fluctuate throughout the day. One study of healthy adults found that the levels of anandamide, one of the two major endocannabinoids, are three times higher after waking up compared to immediately before sleep."[150]

But whatever the reason, there are things to consider before choosing to wake and bake. What do you have planned for the day? Will you be driving any time soon? These answers will tell you if you have the luxury of a slow sipping hippie speedball for breakfast.

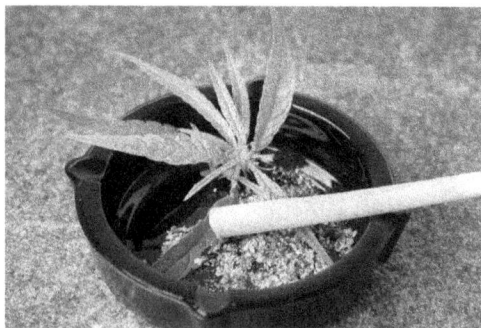

"White Ash Means It's Clean."
This one has been hanging around for decades, and you will still find inconclusive arguments on the topic. The idea is that if the ashes at the end of your joint or in your bowl are white, you have a high quality, clean flower you are smoking on. To find black ashes at the end means you're smoking garbage that may be filled with chemicals or wasn't harvested properly.

One opinion will say that the black or dark gray ash comes from the plant not being "flushed" prior to harvest. "Flushing" is when a grower will only offer the plant clean water in the last few weeks before harvesting to flush out any extra

---

[150]https://cannigma.com/research/wake-and-bake/

nutrients or fertilizers from the soils that the plant has been feeding on.

Another opinion is that the flowers from the plant were not cured (dried) properly, and it is the excess moisture that is to blame for the dark ashes. Much like wood on a campfire, when dry wood is involved, you will get white or light gray ashes at the base of your firepit. But if you were to try to burn wet wood, you end up with coal-like chunks that never fully break down into ashes.

And then there is the role that combustion plays in smoking cannabis. "Research shows that when combustion takes place at a high temperature, organic material is burnt properly leading to a low concentration of nitrogen, and by extension, clear ash colors. On the other hand, when combustion occurs at a low temperature, organic compounds are not properly burnt, thereby leaving a darker ash color."[151]

So, this tells us that the ash color may have everything to do with the temperatures of combustion and not the quality of our flower.

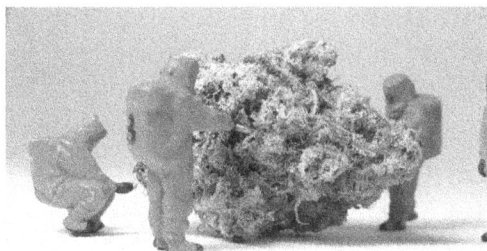

"Weed Hasn't Killed Anyone, So It's Totally Safe."

Ummmm .... No.

This assumption is reckless. To also say that cannabis is a plant, so therefore it is harmless, is another stupid statement. Cocaine comes from a plant. Heroin comes from a plant. Your argument is invalid.

Let's say you took a healthy, middle-aged person with zero medical conditions and they took zero medications; the statement that "no one has died from cannabis," would be true. But realistically, who can check all of those boxes? Just about everyone has something or takes something (including supplements). This opens doors for potential interactions and/or adverse effects which could have grave results. Plus, if you are not growing it yourself there is always the chance that some idiot has used toxic growing practices or has sprayed something ungodly on their products.

---

[151]https://cannabis.net/blog/opinion/cannabis-urban-legend-the-white-ash-vs.-black-ash-myth

---

But in the grand scheme of things of what people can take for either medicinal or recreational purposes, clean cannabis is way, way, way safer than prescriptions, alcohol, or other drugs.

Purple Flower

All right folks, that is quite enough. Stop drinking the purple Kool-Aid! Just because a bud is purple does not mean that it is extra strong or special.

If you are attempting to grow "purps," know that the flower has to have a genetic predisposition for a high concentration of anthocyanins (a group of flavonoids responsible for the colors in fruits and veggies) and it is the environment that coaxes out the color. When your plant is exposed to colder temperatures, the chlorophyll begins to break down and makes room for the color-producing anthocyanins. This is also how we get our amazing fall colors.[152]

So why are people drawn to the purple nugs in display jars? Because they look different—exotic if you will—and those marketing cannabis flower know the general public are suckers for cool packaging (guilty). So, if you insist on using your eyes instead of your nose as your go-to method in choosing a flower, just look for the frosty goodness of the trichomes.

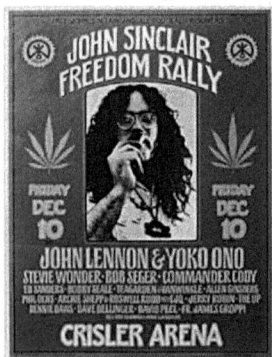

Hash Bash – John Sinclair

The history of the Ann Arbor Hash Bash begins with John Sinclair's possession of two (yes, just two) joints which landed him a ten-year prison sentence in 1969 under Michigan's felony marijuana laws. The December 10, 1971, "John Sinclair Freedom Rally" at Crisler Center arena brought together John Lennon, Yoko Ono, Stevie Wonder, and Bob Seger, among others, to join Sinclair's wife, Leni, in pushing for his release. Sinclair had been in prison for over two years at this point. Lennon even wrote a new song for the occasion, "John Sinclair."

On March 9th, 1972, the Michigan Supreme Court decided that the laws used to convict John Sinclair were unconstitutional, and Michigan legislature changed marijuana possession into a misdemeanor. With a small window of opportunity,

---

[152]https://www.veriheal.com/blog/growing-cannabis/why-turn-purple/

---

as this new classification didn't kick in until April 3rd, the still-anonymous founders suggested they throw a "hash festival" on April Fool's Day to celebrate. They went as far as to claim that such rock stars as Van Morrison would be attending the event. Of course, this wasn't true, but the Michigan Daily picked up the story anyhow. According to the publication 500 people showed up (the police put the number around 150), there were no arrests, and the Ann Arbor News called it an "orderly festival."[153]

As a few months went by, an ordinance was drafted by the Ann Arbor City Council making possession of marijuana a small $5 fine, and the midwestern safe space for cannabis was born.

The very next year, the Hash Bash reported that 5,000 people showed up, including the pro-marijuana legalization State Rep. Perry Bullard, who smiled for the cameras while he was enjoying toking on a joint. As the late '70s and early '80s rolled on, the turnout was less than impressive with it being the "Just Say No" Regan years, but the Hash Bash refused to die.

The Hash Bash crowd rose up to 5,000 again in 1989, and after some legal pushing and shoving between the University of Michigan and the Michigan chapter of NORML, the Hash Bash was moved to the first Saturday in April in 1991, bringing up to 10,000 cannabis supporters to the Diag.

—

The Hash Bash just celebrated its 52nd anniversary in 2023. And as always, it is a welcomed tradition after a long, frigid, sometimes not completely over, Michigan winter. The music, the food, the passionate speakers exercising our freedom of speech, and the simple comradery of partaking publicly outdoors is celebrated.

But hear me and heed me, you still must be aware of your steps in Ann Arbor when it comes to possession. You could be on one side of the street and be protected by the Michigan marijuana laws, as you'll be on state/city land. But if you cross that same street and find yourself on campus (federal) property, you are now poking at a very cranky federal bear.[154]

---

[153]*https://komornlaw.com/some-hash-bash-history/*
[154]*https://dpss.umich.edu/content/prevention-education/safety-tips/alcohol-drugs/marijuana-u-m-faq/*

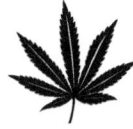

CLOSING

Well, there you have it folks. You now know what I know about cannabis. Maybe my stories made you laugh. Maybe they tugged a bit at your heartstrings. But above all, I hope you have learned something that you didn't know before. Some will say this was too much and others will say that it isn't enough. Both opinions would be correct.

As I bring this book to a close, I'd be willing to bet that more cannabis scientific advances and knowledge has been gained since you started reading. So, I dare you to keep going. I double-dog dare you! Keep learning! Because in the words of Nelson Mandela, "Education is the most powerful weapon which you can use to change the world." And since ignorance is no longer a defense, as you are now an educated consumer, I urge you to learn something new every day. To continue to share your knowledge every day. And I firmly believe that you will be changing the world for the better, every day.

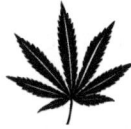

GLOSSARY

Bioavailability: "When a substance such as a medicine or supplement enters your system, the portion of the total substance introduces which can effectively create a response determines that substance's bioavailability. The bioavailability of a substance can fluctuate, depending on the route of administration.

Intravenous administration, or a direct line into the bloodstream, is typically considered 100% bioavailability, as all of the substance will reach target cells. In oral administration routes, AKA when you take a pill, the amount of medicine or supplement you receive depends on many factors, including your diet and your personal metabolism." https://biologydictionary.net/bioavailability/

Blunt: Cannabis flower rolled up in cigar paper and then smoked.

Bong: An apparatus used for smoking cannabis flower using water as a filter. They are generally made from plastic or glass, but can be made using dozens of different materials.

Bowl: An apparatus used for smoking flower. They are generally made from glass but can be made with hundreds of different materials.

Burn One: Smoke a joint.

Cannabis: "The word 'cannabis' refers to all products derived from the plant *Cannabis sativa*" https://www.nccih.nih.gov/health/cannabis-marijuana-and-cannabinoids-what-you-need-to-know

Cannabinoids: "Cannabinoids, broadly speaking, are a class of biological compounds that bind to cannabinoid receptors. They are most frequently sourced from and associated with the plants of the Cannabis genus, including *Cannabis sativa, Cannabis indica*, and *Cannabis ruderalis*." Sheikh NK, Dua A. Cannabinoids. [Updated 2023 Feb 27]. In: StatPearls [Internet]. Treasure Island (FL): StatPearls Publishing; 2023 Jan-. Available from: https://www.ncbi.nlm.nih.gov/books/NBK556062/

CB1 & CB2 Receptors: "The cannabinoid receptors CB1 and CB2 are key components of the human endocannabinoid system, a biological network involved in regulating physiological and cognitive processes. CB1, which is widely distributed throughout the central nervous system, can be activated by some naturally occurring cannabinoids, or through the use of cannabis and related synthetic compounds, resulting in the "high" associated with marijuana … CB2 is mainly expressed in the immune system (to a lesser extent in the central nervous system) and does not create a psychotropic reaction." NIDA. 2019, January 25. A whole new view of CB2. Retrieved from https://nida.nih.gov/news-events/news-releases/2019/01/a-whole-new-view-of-cb2 on 2023, May 21

Chemotypes: "… are often defined by the most abundant chemical produced by that individual and the concept has been useful in work done by chemical ecologists and natural product chemists." https://en.wikipedia.org/wiki/Chemotype

C.O.A or Certificate of Analysis: The test results of the cannabis flower that contains total cannabinoid and/or terpene concentrations.

Concentrate: The end product of condensing the cannabis flower. Other names – Shatter, Wax, crumble, badder, resin, rosin, FECO

Cottonmouth: When your mouth is so dry it feels like cotton.

"Cured": The process of removing moisture from a substance. In curing the cannabis plant, trichomes are degraded and therefore less abundant prior to extraction.

Dab: A hit of concentrate.

Decarboxylation: The process of changing the chemical composition of cannabinoids.

Diamonds/Sand: The end product of crystallized THCA. Diamonds can be crushed to make a sand-like consistency.

Edible: A product that you eat that has cannabis in it.

Endocannabinoids: "The endocannabinoid system (ECS) is a widespread neuromodulatory system that plays important roles in central nervous system (CNS) development, synaptic plasticity, and the response to endogenous and environmental insults. The ECS is comprised of cannabinoid receptors, endogenous cannabinoids (endocannabinoids), and the enzymes responsible for the synthesis and degradation of the endocannabinoids." Lu HC, Mackie K. An Introduction to the Endogenous Cannabinoid System. Biol Psychiatry. 2016 Apr 1;79(7):516-25. doi: 10.1016/j.biopsych.2015.07.028. Epub 2015 Oct 30. PMID: 26698193; PMCID: PMC4789136.

Flavonoids: "Currently there are about 6000 flavonoids that contribute to the colourful pigments of fruits, herbs, vegetables and medicinal plants." Iwashina T. Contribution to flower colors of flavonoids including anthocyanins: a review. Nat Prod Commun. 2015 Mar;10(3):529-44. PMID: 25924543.

FECO: Fully Extracted Cannabis Oil.

Flower: The sticky buds found on the cannabis plant that are covered in the trichomes that contain cannabinoids, terpenes, and flavonoids.

Other names – reefer, devils' lettuce, weed, dope, pot, ganja, herb, grass, Mary Jane, Kush, kind, chronic

Negative names – boof, ditch weed, brick weed, mids, Reggie, schwag, bunk

Genotype: Genotypes are the DNA or blueprint of that particular cannabis plant, its genetic makeup, or genetic potential if you will.

Hemp/Industrial Hemp: "Is a botanical class of *Cannabis sativa* cultivars grown specifically for industrial or medicinal use. It can be used to make a wide range of products.[1] Along with bamboo, hemp is among the fastest growing plants[2] on Earth. It was also one of the first plants to be spun into usable fiber 50,000 years ago.[3] It can be refined into a variety of commercial items, including paper, rope, textiles, clothing, biodegradable plastics, paint, insulation, biofuel, food, and animal feed." https://en.wikipedia.org/wiki/Hemp

Joint: Cannabis flower rolled up in paper and then smoked like a cigarette.

Other names – jay, fatty, left-handed cigarette(lefty), and doobie

Kief: The trichomes that have been knocked off of the cannabis flower. Sometimes collected in the bottom compartment of a flower grinder.

Landrace: A genetically pure cannabis plant.

"Live": Refers to when a cannabis plant is directly flash frozen at harvest. This preserves more of the trichomes prior to extraction.

Marijuana: "The word 'marijuana' refers to parts of or products from the plant *Cannabis sativa* that contain substantial amounts of tetrahydrocannabinol (THC)." https://www.nccih.nih.gov/health/cannabis-marijuana-and-cannabinoids-what-you-need-to-know

Moon rocks: A bud rolled in hash oil and then rolled in kief or bubble/ice water hash.

Oil: Can refer to tincture, cartridges, or concentrates.

Phenotype: When a genotype is exposed to the environment (temps, altitude, indoor or out), and the end result will be your phenotype.

Phytocannabinoids: "... a molecule synthesized by plants. There are 113 known phytocannabinoids in the cannabis plant." https://foliumbiosciences.com/what-is-a-phytocannabinoid/

Pen: the battery for vape cartridges or concentrates.

Pinner: A small joint. Usually rolled too tight.

Puff, Puff, Pass: Means you are taking too long with your turn when smoking in groups.

Purge: The process of flushing or clearing a cannabis plant of solvents used in the extraction process.

Roach: The remains of a smoked joint.

Rig: An apparatus used for smoking concentrates. They can be heated using a blowtorch or an electric hook up.

RSO: Rick Simpson Oil

Sauce: Liquid terpenes that are added to concentrates for added flavor and effects.

Skins: Rolling papers.

Spliff: A mix of cannabis flower and tobacco rolled up and smoked.

Stepped On: When another substance is added to dilute the original product.

Sublingual: Latin for "under the tongue."

Tarantula Leg: A joint rolled in hash oil and then rolled in kief or bubble/ice water hash.

Terpenes: "… the largest and most diverse group of naturally occurring compounds that are mostly found in plants but larger classes of terpenes such as sterols and squalene can be found in animals. They are responsible for the fragrance, taste, and pigment of plants." "The common plant sources of terpenes are tea, thyme, cannabis, Spanish sage, and citrus fruits (e.g., lemon, orange, mandarin)." Cox-Georgian D, Ramadoss N, Dona C, Basu C. Therapeutic and Medicinal Uses of Terpenes. Medicinal Plants. 2019 Nov 12:333–59. doi: 10.1007/978-3-030-31269-5_15. PMCID: PMC7120914.

Tincture: "… a solution of a medicinal substance in an alcoholic solvent." https://www.merriam-webster.com/dictionary/tincture

Total Cannabinoids: The complete number of all of the cannabinoids that appear in test results.

Trichomes: "Trichomes are shoot epidermal hairs, found on the majority of plants, and are composed of either single or several cells (Esau, 1977). They play various protective roles, such as being a mechanical barrier to insect herbivores, filtering UV light and reducing respiration." (Fordyce and Agrawal, 2001; Karabourniotis *et al.*, 1992; Levin, 1973; Ripley *et al.*, 1999; Van Dam and Hare,1998).

CORRECTION AND RETRACTION POLICY

I. Introduction
The integrity of my content is of utmost importance regarding the published *Pot for the People* and the "Budtenders Blueprint" training. This Correction and Retraction Policy outlines the procedure to address mistakes, inaccuracies, or misleading information that may be discovered in our publications, products, or services.

II. Corrections
A. Minor Corrections: *

1. Spelling, Grammar, Punctuation: These corrections will be made promptly without formal notice.

2. Factual Errors: If a minor factual error is detected, the mistake will be corrected, and a note will be appended to the corrected content, clearly stating the nature and date of the correction.

B. Major Corrections: *

1. Significant Factual Errors or Misinterpretations: Corrections will be made, and a formal correction notice will be issued alongside the content, clearly explaining the nature and date of the correction.

III. Retractions
A. Grounds for Retraction: *

1. Plagiarism

2. Fraudulent or Fabricated Data

3. Ethical Misconduct

B. Retraction Procedure:

1. Investigation: The issue will be thoroughly investigated by the responsible team or committee.

2. Decision: A decision to retract will be made in consultation with key stakeholders, such as authors, editors, or legal advisors.

3. Notification: Affected parties will be notified of the decision.

4. Public Notice: A retraction notice will be published, clearly stating the reason for retraction and the nature of the offense.

IV. Transparency

All corrections and retractions will be handled with full transparency, and all involved parties will be informed as necessary.

V. Contact Information

For questions or to report a concern, please contact:

Angela Roullier

potforthepeople.co@gmail.com

www.ingramcontent.com/pod-product-compliance
Lightning Source LLC
Chambersburg PA
CBHW052112020426

42335CB00021B/2724